Living with ADHD

Chris Fife
© 12/30/14

Table of Contents

Introduction

Many teachers and parents are no strangers to ADHD (attention deficit hyperactive disorder). It has been diagnosed for thousands of children and adults. The big question is its causes and the treatments for it. For many who live with this disorder it can be very difficult to do anything that requires focus and concentration. This includes sitting still in a classroom, reading, and listening to others. It can drive parents, teachers, and other people who do not understand it crazy.

This book is an attempt to bring some light to ADHD from a non-clinical point of view. What is it like to live with ADHD as both a child and an adult? What caused me to get ADHD? How can I deal with it and have a normal life? It can be a scary journey for parents and children, but it can also be something that is manageable and can even be exciting.

Today more than ever before people are living with ADHD. Whether you believe it is diet, lifestyle, pollution, or genetics ADHD has a huge impact on many people's lives. It is important to be able to understand it and learn how to live with it.

Chapter One: A Rough Childhood

When I was growing up, I was always in the lowest math, and English class. I had a hard time pronouncing words, and I did not like to read, because I had a hard time reading. I remember one year my parents were talking about that I might have to be held back a grade, because I was not doing well in school. In elementary school, because I did not do well, I was teased and bullied a lot, which lead me to be very sad and depressed.

At the time it was in the 1970's and the only advice for someone like me was to buck up and do my best. My mother would force me to read each night yelling at me if I did not read correctly and making me struggle with all of the painful words I had to try to pronounce. My parents were supportive in the only way they knew and that was that I just needed to do everything I was told to do and work hard at it. Even if I tried as hard as I could and did not do well I was told I was stupid.

I did not do much to get into trouble. So there was that part of my life that I was saved from, but there was still plenty to make me have a poor self esteem, and feel sad all of the time. For a time the school put me in resource with a speech therapist. This helped a little, but I still had a hard time reading and concentrating in school. I liked to day dream and think about the future.

I remember that when Star Wars came out, I thought of all of these stories that I could write about Star Wars. It was a shame that I was not a good writer at the time, or I would have been able to have capitalized on all of the money the Star Wars books have taken in. My mind was very active and I had a very active imagination thinking about all sorts of things that would be considered science fiction or fantasy.

I remember coming up with an idea about vampires from outer space, and that I was part of this race of people that came from a distant galaxy. In part a lot of my imagination involved escaping my life, because I was miserable and wanted to be someone else. For a time I wanted to be Elvis Presley who at the time was the most famous person I knew. I thought of being a great singer and actor. The only problem was I couldn't sing or act and was too scared to even talk with people.

I had developed a phobia of talking with people to the point that I never said anything in my classes and spoke little to friends at school even during recess and lunch. I felt alone like I had no friends and that no one at my school liked me. There were a few times I remember doing foolish things to get the attention of other students. I drank three or four small milk cartons very fast. I walked around a small island during the winter in the park in water that had both ice on top and ice in the bottom. I slipped in the water and got all wet and cold from the experience. I sang songs to a girl I liked, I fought a kid, because the other kids wanted me to. There were numerous times when I did things just because I wanted attention and wanted people to know that I was alive.

There were even times when I thought that if I would only die and then people would feel sorry for me and morn over me, because I was dead. I had a lot of thoughts of suicide back then, because of all of what was happening to me. It was a tough time in my life, and even over forty years later, I still have problems talking to people and difficulty reading and socializing with people.

At the time, I thought I was just a normal kid who was just having a tough time. I hated myself and hated that I was stupid, but I thought that this was just the way I was and I just had to live with this. I withdrew and became shy and mentally checked out and allowed my imagination to take over and became consumed with television. We first only had one television and I would watch just what my parents wanted to watch at night. This was not too exciting, but I did see it as an escape from reality. Then we got two television sets, and at the time there were no cell phones, and the computers were no better than word processors and calculators. The internet did not exist either, so the only media release I had was television, and when we got the second television it meant that me and my sisters could watch what we wanted to watch and when my sisters were not watching television, I could watch what I wanted to watch.

This did not mean that we had over 200 channels to choose from. It meant that we had 5 channels, the main three and the two PBS channels we received over our antenna. At the time PBS just showed boring documentaries and things for grown ups which left me with three channels and a certain time period to watch television at. I worked it out that when I got home from school, I would watch a couple hours of children's programming and then watch what my sisters wanted to watch for a couple hours at night. We would take a break at 6:00 when the news came on and then finish our night in front of the television.

I do not remember doing a lot of homework those days, a lot of it was watching television. I believe I did the homework, because my mother would get mad at me if I didn't get it done. But for the most part I watched a lot of television, including waking up at 5:00 Saturday morning to watch cartoons especially my favorite which was Hong Kong Fuii. There were times when I would wake up my sisters and they would get mad at me so I attempted to watch it with the volume really low.

At the time I did not realize what was happening in my life, but there was a definite pattern developing. I had a creative imagination, but it was not leading me anywhere and at the time my parents whenever I said something like I wanted to be a professional singer, athlete, or artist they would just look at me as if I was an alien and tell me I was crazy. Then at school none of the teachers ever encouraged me to go into anything I liked and I was not good at anything else in school, so I thought my life was hopeless. My imagination was only an outlet for me to escape my reality, it was not until I was older that I realized that my imagination could have done so much more for me.

I sunk into the pattern of allowing media to be part of my imagination with all of the television series that I had watched. The ones I liked the most were science fiction like Buck Rogers, Battlestar Galactica, and Star Trek the Next Generation. My mind would wonder to these programs and I envisioned being part of them. There was one show called Grizzly Adams where a man goes to live in the mountains with the animals. I associated with him and wanted to live in the mountains like he did. So I ran away from home and was on my way to the mountains when my parents picked me up. I ended up going home and watching Grizzly Adams wondering what it would have been like if I would have been able to have gone to the mountains.

I also started to develop a way of thinking like the adults around me that I just had to be tough and do what I was told to do. I thought that it was just about hard work and that if I was stupid I just had to work harder at being better. No one considered that I might have had a learning disability. Back then a learning disability generally meant something severe like Downs Syndrome or something mild like a speak impediment which I was treated for. But when it came to mainstream learning disabilities like dyslexia and ADHD these were virtually unknown at the time.

Instead of telling me I had a learning disability, I was told that I was lazy and stupid. The problem is that when you are told you are something for a long enough time you become what everyone tells you who you are. I thought I was lazy and stupid and so I acted the part. I had given up with attempting to tell my parents and teachers that there was something wrong, because they would just continue to tell me that I just needed to work harder and not be lazy. It was hard enough to convince my parents that I was allergic to eggs.

The conversation would go as follows, "I have cooked some eggs for you for breakfast," my father told me.

"I can't eat the eggs, I am allergic to them," I said back.

"Oh, yeah that's right you do not like eggs, but I made them for you and they will go to waste," my father told me.

"But I can't eat them, I am allergic to them and they will make me sick if I eat them," I tried to explain.

"Okay, fine, I guess I will have to eat them," he yelled at me.

Then a few months later the same situation would happen. But eventually my parents would just not fix eggs for me, but not because I was allergic to them, it was because they thought I just did not like eggs. It was as if they did not even pay attention to what I was telling them. When I was younger, I loved eggs and eat a lot of them, it wasn't until I was older that I had developed an allergic reaction to them. But even for years my parents and older sister always just thought I did not like eggs and couldn't understand that I was allergic to them.

The same thing happened when I tried to convince them that I was having a hard time concentrating at school and did not know what the teacher was talking about. It was hard for me to explain to my parents what I was going through, so I gave up trying and just struggled through school and life hoping for the best.

I always thought that the best was right around the corner and I would be able to have the American dream. I thought about going to high school and how I would be able to be popular and have girl friends. Then I would be a professional football player or body builder and make enough money to have the house of my dreams and to be able to get married and have a family. It was something that I thought was a natural thing that happened to everyone, that they just waited and their dreams came true. I knew that I would have to work hard at exercise in order to get my dream to come true, but I didn't understand just how hard I would have to work, and that there would be a lot of obstacles in my way.

I managed to get through elementary school and went to junior high school. This was exciting because with junior high meant that I could play school sports and I could take P.E. and art class two classes I ended up taking every year until I graduated from high school. I ended up liking junior high better than elementary, because there were more students I could see and more teachers. I fell right into the grove of things and my parents even said that if I got good grades they would give me money.

I was still very shy and would even get sick if I had to answer the phone or was in a situation where I had to talk with someone, and I still had a hard time concentrating on my schoolwork and reading. In elementary school I only remember reading one book *The Adventures of Robinson Cruiso*. There were other books, but not a lot, and in junior high I also did not read. I got into the habit of being able to read just enough out of my text books to be able to pass my classes, but I had never just read a text book cover to cover.

When I read a book my mind begins to wonder, and it becomes difficult for me to concentrate on what I am reading. I often would read ten pages and did not know what I just read. It was difficult at best to concentrate on reading and be able to understand what I read. It wasn't until I read Arnold Swarzzeneger's *Education of a Bodybuilder* that I was able to read a book cover to cover and understand everything I just read. It also got me excited about reading book, body building books. I was able to read several of these books, but for the average book it took me months to read. The body building books only took me a few weeks to read. I had learned that when I was excited about something I was able to do it in far less time and was able to do it better than I did other things.

The only problem was that body building was not in the curriculum at school. The only thing that came close was P.E. class and this did not help me in math or English. I still had a hard time in these classes and struggled in my classes to do well. I am not sure what happened, but I suddenly was able to start doing well in my classes, by just showing up every day on time and doing all of the homework and work in class. I still had a hard time understanding the teacher, but by doing the work I was able do.

The end result was that I was able to pass all of my classes, and started to even get better with my grades, eventually getting on the honor role and getting straight A's one quarter. Only I was not really a straight A student and I just did well because I got to know what the teacher wanted and then turned in all of my assignments.

In high school I took all of the easy classes and finished school with a 3.5 GPA. There was a time I was doing okay in English even though I still didn't read a lot of books and had a hard time reading, and I managed to do well in math, except when my family moved to another state where I failed Geometry because it was a different school, a different teacher, and a different book they were going through all a combination of failure waiting to happen. Yet through it all I continued to struggle to concentrate and learn what was being taught.

Exercise helped me to focus better, and I felt a lot better when I exercised, but when I was not exercising I was daydreaming and watching television. This was my world, and there was no direction in it to lead to success. Sure there was high school graduation, but I did not want to go to college. The only thing left was to get a job and the jobs I wanted were so far out there it would have been better for me if I would have attempted to go to the moon. I had lofty dreams and no understanding of how to get there.

When I got to high school there was no guidance, and the counselor just talked to me about my schedule. They did not tell me about college entrance exams, or what I needed to do to get into college, but then again I did not want to go to college. So I might have missed some of the extra things they offered students like talking about a future in college. There was not as many opportunities back then like there are now, I wasn't able to attend college early, take concurrent classes, or take classes at the ATC. At the time, I am not sure I would have seized the opportunity to take any of those classes, because I had developed an attitude that I hated school, and once I was finished with high school, I was done with school.

Looking back at my childhood, I can start to understand what I was going through and why I had such a hard time at school. It wasn't until years later, I suddenly realized that I have ADHD, or at least some form of it. I have never been diagnosed as having ADHD, but I have a lot of what would be considered the symptoms of it.

As a teacher I was in a conference listening to a specialist from the district talking to a student of mine and his parents. She was explaining to the student and the parents what it was like to have ADHD. I suddenly realized that everything she was saying I experienced, especially when she mentioned that a person with ADHD has a difficult time reading and comprehending the material because his mind is too busy. I knew then that I had ADHD, and that all my life I have struggled with it.

When I hated reading as a child it was because I had a hard time reading and understanding what I read. I got so that I would be able to read out loud okay. But when I read silently I had a hard time focusing on what I read and my mind would wonder off. It took me twenty minutes to read one page in a book and nearly a year to finish the book, and then when I finished the book, I could not remember anything that I had just read.

It was not just reading either, I had a hard time listening and understanding my teachers. They would explain something like a math problem and I would not be able to concentrate on what they were saying and then my mind would be distracted by my thoughts and I would drift into day dreaming about something. At the time, I didn't realize it but my mind was like that of a fictional writer coming up with stories all of the time. Terry Brooks described this in his book about writing as the way he thought. He said that he would go to dinner with some friends and while they were talking he would suddenly drift off and think about some story line. I was the same way, and this not only effected my reading and listening to the teacher, but it affected my social life as well.

I am shy by nature, and this was why I did not do a lot of social things when I was growing up like going to a lot of dances. Yet it was also something more, I was easily distracted when I was around other people, and had a hard time following someone's conversation and getting into the conversation. My mind would wonder and I would think about other things, and then when I thought of something and got the opportunity to share it, my friends would look at me and think I was a little crazy, because what I said was completely different than what they were talking about, and some of what I would say was out there more fictional than reality.

It is another reason why I did not go on a lot of dates, because I could not have a normal conversation. When my family moved to Ohio when I was in 10th grade there were several girls who did not know me, and I was able to ask them out on a date, but after one date they did not want to go out with me anymore. In part because I was a space case thinking about other things than thinking about what was happening, or that I was thinking too much about what was happening and was so nervous that it was like taking a final exam. I was nervous and uncomfortable the entire time on my date, and my date could tell that I was too serious and this was something they did not like.

The essence of my childhood was that I had a hard time with several things in school, at home, and among friends, and I believe because I had ADHD and at the time it was something that was still just being looked at and researched. I didn't even hear about it until after I had graduated from high school, and got into teaching. Even if someone would have suggested I had it when I was younger and got me tested, they would not have known what to do with me. By the time I was in high school, I was passing all of my classes and doing a good job of it. But life would have been a lot better, if I knew what I was dealing with and worked on being able to control it.

Another thing that had bothered me is how I got it. What caused me to have ADHD? I had heard that it could be in part genetic, and my father is proof that he could have passed some of his ADHD to me. He did okay growing up, but never really read much, and he had to constantly be moving around. My dad also liked to watch a lot of television, and both my grandfathers watched a lot of television as well. Both of whom did not have a college degree and struggled as readers. So I can say that I definitely have had a genetic disposition for ADHD and I also see it in my daughter as well.

The other thing I believe contributed to my ADHD was watching a lot of television. People may argue that technology does not have anything to do with ADHD, but I know that television, video games, texting and spending time on the internet stimulates the brain and forms connections which in turn could make the brain more active and harder to control. Television combined with my imagination caused my brain to work overtime to form connections. This could be a good thing if I can control my thoughts because it means that my brain can come up with a lot of different ideas. It is just a matter of applying those ideas to life. It was not often the inventor who became rich off of their invention, but the guy later who came along and make the idea affordable and available to the public.

The other thing that contributed to my ADHD was going through traumatic events. I did not go through very terrible things like Martin Luther King III had gone through. He described how in his book he had ADHD and it was because of all of the things his family went through for the civil rights movement which can to a peak with the death of his father. I did go through relentless teasing in school, and was told by kids, teachers, and my parents that I was a loser, stupid, and good for nothing. I believe that it was my depression that caused my brain to come up with a defense mechanism which allowed me to escape with my fantasies. I got so good at daydreaming that I could picture anyone in my mind and act out a story in my mind.

My active imagination not only followed my daydreaming, it came out in my dreams too. I have always had vivid dreams where I could do just about anything including be the hero of my dream. I was always picturing me as the hero who could do just about anything to save the day and help the people I cared about. I was also the hero of the community and at school where all of the kids would look at me and say, "Look there goes Chris Fife, he saved our lives."

So with the depression, the heredity, television, and a poor diet, I am convinced those things helped to contribute to my ADHD. There was little to do with me being able to change my heritage, but I could have changed the other three. I could have limited or eliminated my television viewing. Ate better food and got control over my depression. I also know that if I would have been able to have had the support of family, friends, and the school I would have provided some services.

By accident I did learn some things that helped me tremendously with controlling my ADHD. The first was exercise, it helped me to focus better and it gave me the discipline in order to be able to get to school and to my classes on time as well as doing all of the work including homework. The other thing that helped me was to realize that I could focus on the things I was most interested at the time. As an example, I got excited about body building for a time, so I read all of the books about body building that I could and got really into it. The more excited about something I got the better focus and direction my brain was heading in.

I was fortunate to have survived my childhood and graduate from college and later get a master's degree. There were times, however, that I was so depressed I could have easily gotten a more serious mental illness, or have taken my life. There was the time I ran away from home, and if successful could have been on the streets, or in the mountains and would have probably had died of exposure to the elements. I also at one point seriously considered dropping out of school all together and just got a job.

There were people around me as supports, but I was unaware of them, and refused to seek the help that I desperately needed. It was a catch 22 where I was shy and was too scared to ask for help, but I needed the help to overcome a lot of what I was going through. I was reluctant to ask my parents for help, because they were difficult to talk with and I was scared of talking to them especially when it came to getting help for school.

I decided to write this book to go through what I did to survive ADHD and as an adult what I do to live with ADHD. In many cases children outgrow a lot of the symptoms, but there are a few who continue on with ADHD into adulthood and I was one of them. I struggled with it through college, and at work as a teacher. I am faced with the same challenges as an adult as I had when I was a child. I still have a hard time reading and understanding things, and I still have a hard time staying focused when someone is talking to me. One thing I am surprised at is that there are a lot of teachers who had ADHD. I am not sure if it is a good thing, but they can at least relate to some of their students like I have been able to.

I was able to live with ADHD for nearly forty years and have been successful in my life. In this book I would like to share some of the things that have helped me deal with my ADHD. I hope that they will be beneficial and help in understanding how ADHD affects our lives and what we can do to overcome some of the negative effects of ADHD. Read this book with an open mind and use it as a guide for some of the things you or someone you know can follow in balancing their lives and gaining the success they want.

Chapter Two: Causes and Symptoms of ADHD

In order to control something in your life, you need to understand it. Many people still do not understand ADHD especially those who have it, and therefore it is not only difficult to diagnose and it is difficult to treat as well. Child psychologists receive more training than anyone else when it comes to ADHD, and then there are those who have studied it and the affects it has on children. But there has not been a lot of study, research, and training on adult ADHD, and overall ADHD has been the least studied of many mental disorders. Some would even argue that it doesn't exist as a disorder.

When I first became a teacher I heard about it, and thought that it was something made up by doctors in order to be able to make money, and that children did not have to take drugs they just needed to quit being lazy and just start doing the work. Even as a teacher having several students with ADHD, I denied that it really existed and thought that it was a shame that these children were being doped up in order to be able to function in school. I thought that children were being over medicated and abused with medications.

Yet when looking at ADHD there is a definite pattern involved with the symptoms and the treatment that work together. In my own life I have experienced a distracted mind where at times it is difficult to concentrate especially when it comes to things that I am bored with. My mind can get bored easily, and at school when I was in a math class where I did not understand the teacher, I just took a nap each day I was in class. This was counterproductive because I failed the class and the teacher probably thought I was a lazy kid who should not have been in his class. I can also understand that he had a full class and was probably doing all that he could to just teach the material and did not have time to worry about a new kid to his class who just slept all of the time and got zeros on the quizzes and assignments.

I did not want to fail the class and wanted to be able to get the credit for math, but I was stressed out because my parents had just moved to another state in a new school, and I was scared of the teachers, the classes, and the students. I had just been walking outside around the buildings during lunch at the school and the police officer at the school got mad at me, because he told me I could not do that and the school was a closed campus. This upset me and I didn't think I could do anything right at the school.

So when my math teacher got up and gave his lesson on how to do the math problems it was as if he was talking in a foreign language I did not know anything about. I was taking Spanish at the time and knew more about what was happening in my Spanish class then I did in my math class, and the Spanish teacher taught most of his lessons in Spanish. I was not sure why I did not know anything about what the math teacher was talking about, because I was doing fine at my other school and got A's in math the year before. But it was as if I had missed more than a half a year in my math class and needed the foundation to be able to pass the class, and my brain was so blocked by distractions that I could not focus or be able to figure out what was going on.

As a teacher with nearly 50 percent of students not passing math classes at the school I teach at there is something going on. I have also heard that most college freshmen cannot pass college math and have to take it three times before they are able to pass it. Yet there are some students who have ADHD who excel in math, but have a hard time in language arts. I believe it has to do with the stress level they have in those classes and their own personal interest. I did not do well in math because I was stressed out and had no interest in math.

My parents had be get tutored in math after I failed third term in math, and with one on one tutoring going through the beginning of the text book, I was able to pick up the math, only my class was at the end of the book doing things I still did not understand. So by the time I was almost caught up with my class the year was over and I received a D-. I was able to do a little better in math the next year, but not that much, and ever since I have had a tough time in my math class, I have had a poor attitude when it comes to math and with this attitude it is hard for me to study math anymore without having anxiety. Even now when I am writing this, I am having some anxiety just thinking about it.

The inability to focus because of distraction is a key to ADHD. Some children exhibit hyperactivity where they just cannot stay still for more than a minute, but again part of the reason is that their mind gets bored and they have to do something to entertain it which means walking around bugging other people, or in the case in a classroom where students are expected to be in their seats they might be spitting spit wads or throwing pencils at other students. It could be that they are teasing or bullying other students as well. For these students this behavior is normal to them, but for others around them it is not the norm and they get upset with the students and they are then in trouble and get upset and agree for getting into trouble for something they believe to be normal and that in their minds there is nothing wrong with it.

The distraction or lack of focus is what often causes the trouble for those with ADHD especially when it might involve education, work, and family relationships. Parents may be upset with their child because she isn't doing what they asked her to do. My daughter whose seven years old explained it in this way, "Dad, I can't concentrate on cleaning my room, I get distracted by playing in my room. I need help."

I knew that she was telling the truth because when we asked her to clean her room an hour later I would find her just playing in her room without having cleaned any of it. Yet with the proper motivation she was able to finish it either through not being able to play with friends or giving her a reward for doing it like some money. Yet this was not the right way to handle the situation. I always want to do things the quickest and easiest way, so I do the reward or punishment practice as a parent which does not teach my daughter how to handle her emotions and concentrate on the task at hand. The proper way to handle the situation would be to talk her through cleaning her room and teach her how to recognize when she is getting bored and for her to come back to the task at hand. I struggle with this as well when I get off take it is difficult to come back to what I am doing.

I have heard that the ADHD mind is like a fast car that has no brakes. Another analogy is that the mind is like a tree where birds are flying from one branch to the next. The tree is the brain and the birds are thoughts. In an ADHD mind the birds are flying back and forth to the point of confusion. There is also the idea that the mind is like a stage and the thought come across the stage and you invite thoughts to come across the stage of your mind and choose which ones you want to allow to remain on the stage. Another one is that thoughts are like plants and you can either reject the plants or you can let them take root in your mind.

While I was sitting in the living room, I thought about my mind as being in a living room and people coming to my house and entering the living room. The people represent thoughts in my mind and start to have conversations with me. The only problem is that every person in the living room has their own agenda and things to say about something completely different. The living room can get crowded at times and it is difficult for me to think and process my thoughts. I go from one person to another having a conversation with them attempting to satisfy the person's need. I have thoughts about work, personal interest, or family that will come into my mind and I will give it some of my attention, but then I will go to something else, and the previous thought remains in my mind until my mind is satisfied with the attention I give to it.

When I allow my imagination to take place it consumes my mind to the point all other thoughts are removed, and I am left to my fantasy that I have created. It can sometimes be my sanctuary a place of refuge from all of the stress of life and a place where I am able to express myself and be myself. Yet the fantasy that my mind explores causes me to ignore those thoughts in my mind that need my attention and if there is something important that I need to focus on it becomes difficult at best to be able to work that out.

The best way to deal with my thoughts were to invite them into the living room understand what they want and then dismiss the ones that are not worthy of the time and effort I would give it and focus on the most urgent ones that need my attention like financial issues in paying bills or family issues about upcoming events. It could also be work related that cannot wait.

The symptoms then can be somewhat troublesome if they distract you from doing what you would like to do. It can take you twice as long to do things as it would without ADHD. This is why so many students have a hard time with school, is that the classes move in a steady pace according to the curriculum given for the class, and students who are unable to keep up fall behind, and for a student with ADHD if he falls behind it is nearly impossible to catch up with the class.

As an adult I have found that normal mundane tasks like cleaning the house, mowing the lawn, or taking care of the car can take a lot of time to do, and I will purposefully postpone some of these tasks because I think of them as boring, even though I know that I will have to do them eventually. This causes a lot of problems for me, because I will then have several tasks to do that will pile up at home. I do the same things with my stuff that I get in the mail, or things I am working on.

My desk is cluttered with several different things I am working on or items that I like to use. But there is no organization going on, it is just piles of clutter, and eventually I will go through and clean my desk area, but more times than not my wife will get frustrated with me and clean it for me, unfortunately there is a system I have with all of the chaos and when my wife cleans my desk or my piles of things I then suddenly cannot find the things I had on my desk, because in my mind I remember the general location of where I put my things, and when those things are organized I then cannot find where the things are.

Sometimes I am able to get a system of organizing my things for a while, but then I get bored with it and start to resort back to the chaos of creating piles. I do a similar thing at my school when I am teaching classes. I have never been organized to have lesson plans for what I am teaching. I call it improvisation. I just have a general idea of what I am going to teach and what I want the students to do and then I teach the students what to do.

In my mind I am saving a lot of time not organizing all of my things on my desk and making lesson plans for school. I am not sure if this is the right way to do things, but I have developed a style of being able to make it work for me. When I get into organizing things it seems to take much longer to do, and then I get frustrated with the process and then when I am organized I get bored with it and have a need to change it.

The same thing happens when I teach, I will write up a lesson plan and feel comfortable with what I have done, and then when I teach it, I find myself changing it and doing my own thing. I have a hard time following a lesson plan especially when it comes to my classes and the material I teach. There may be great teaching moments that necessitate deviation from a lesson plan. I know that many people who encounter this type of teaching style or the management style I have would get upset and wonder how I can even function this way.

I have found that I am able to function according to things I have developed over the years in order to live with my ADHD. There are times when I have to conform to my wife's wishes, or my boss's mandate. But it is hard to be able to live by such restrictions and constraints when my mind is going all over the place, and I have a desperate need for liberty of expression and thoughts. Without this freedom my frustration level rises and I have an increased level of distraction which makes it harder to teach, harder to find things at home, and harder for me to function as a good husband and father.

Even writing this book you may find me diverging to something because my thoughts go somewhere else and I come up with something great in my mind that I want to write even though it may not fit exactly into the book. It just takes patience and an open mind when you are dealing with someone with ADHD. If you have ADHD it takes patience, and open mind, and a willingness to do what is necessary for family, job, country, and God.

When it comes to symptoms for ADHD it could be a variety of things such as a learning disability which makes it difficult for you to read or concentrate on your studies. The mind becomes bored easily with things and you will be constantly seeking new things. When I read books I will often read more than one book at a time, because I get bored easily.

Chapter Three: My Way

It is not uncommon that those with ADHD do things their own way and have a hard time conforming to what other people tell them to do. This is why many children with ADHD have a battle with their teachers at their school. It is not that people with ADHD are combative or rebel against authority, it is just that they do not understand the instructions and will be scared to ask for help or clarification.

I am not sure if it is the Scottish blood in me or the way I was raised with my father having his way of doing things, but I have a strong compulsion to do things my way. I am open to suggestions and hear what people have to say, but in the end I have to do it my way, or I go crazy, this is in part to the way my brain is working and how it is constantly moving faster than the speed of light.

It drove me insane some of the things my father had me do while I was growing up, and in part I do the same as a father. One of the jobs I had when I was a kid was to mow the lawn. I would just mow the lawn going back and forth in rows or go around in a circle until I couldn't go in a circle anymore. Sometimes I would get bored and attempt to mow my name into the lawn or do different shapes and designs. In the end, however, I would make sure to have the lawn mowed to my father's perfection.

If I mowed the lawn before my father got home from work, or when he was gone on Saturday, I was lucky and be able to mow the lawn the way I wanted, and I would be able to get the job done faster. But if my father was home he would watch over me as I mowed the lawn like a guard at a high security prison. Immediately I was stressed out and my progress in mowing the lawn would slow done because of the stress and wondering if I was doing it right. Once I got started mowing the lawn, I tried to mow it the way I intended ignoring my father, because of the noise of the lawnmower. But he managed to yell over the lawn mower and even come out and physically grab the lawnmower from my hands and yell, "No you need to do it this way," he then would proceed to show me how to go back and forth over the lawn.

This confused me since, I thought that mowing the lawn was mowing the lawn and there isn't any special way to mow the lawn. You just cut the lawn, and the lawn grows, and you cut it again the following week. I did not see how cutting the lawn one way was any different than cutting it another way, and if my father wasn't home when I cut the lawn he really didn't notice the difference. There is a slight difference in how the lawn would look, but my father never said anything. I also thought he should have been happy that I was even mowing the lawn, and that I was not a rebellious kid who went off with gangs, broke the law, and did drugs.

But there was something in my father's mind that things had to be done his way, and he also had a tendency to want to teach me how to do things perfect, which was his way of doing things. Only this made me hate the idea of perfectionism that is one reason why I hate to do things over again so that it can be perfect, because I had enough of it when I was growing up. All through college I only edited a couple of papers that I had turned in. 99 percent of the papers I had turned in were my first draft, which most people commonly call a rough draft, but I would call my final copy.

Back to what I would call the lawn experiment, I would sometimes have to mow the lawn twice because I was doing it wrong, or because my father thought it needed to be mowed again the opposite way so it would grow better. Later in my life I somehow understood that people do mow their lawns a certain way, because they say it will look better or grow better. I am not sure about that. When I bought a house of my own and did my own lawn experiment on mowing the lawn and even mowing it twice in the opposite direction and on an angle to attempt to make it look like the wealthy homes in the area with green well manicured lawns, I found it didn't look any different than if I mowed it once in a circle, or by rows, or by wavy lines.

Then there was the trimming when I grew up. We did not have an electric or gas powered trimmer for the lawn, we had hand clippers that would bend the grass not cut it because they were so dull. My father made me sit out for hours clipping the lawn, especially the part of the lawn that was only a foot wide next to the fence of our neighbor. I found it was easier to just pull the grass with my hands to the length of what it should have been. I often had blisters every week from trimming the lawn. Later my father bought an electric trimmer which help tremendously in trimming up the lawn, however, he still insisted on me using the hand trimmers on several areas of the lawn, because he felt that the electric one did not do as good of a job. I personally did not see the difference.

To this day, I hate lawns. I hate cutting lawns, trimming lawns, fertilizing lawns, watering lawns, and all of the hard work spent on taking care of something I hate. I do not even like looking or walking on lawns. As a home owner, I feel that lawns are one of the biggest wastes of money for the home. I know that in a given year I could spend over $200.00 to just maintain the lawn. This is a high price to pay for something I despise. Some people might even spend over a thousand dollars a year just to see a green carpet out of their windows. Living in the west it is also insane how much water is wasted watering lawns.

You can see how just something as simple as mowing the lawn can be made into a big deal with ADHD. You see my father was obsessed with doing it just right, and now I hate everything about it, and only do it out of compliance with city ordinances and tradition of having a green weed free lawn. I always wonder why I have to mow the lawn when in nature the grass is left to grow to its normal height. If I were to just let it grow and then buy some goats to eat up the grass then everything would work out.

There were several obsessive things in my childhood that I had to do my father's way. Such as taking a shower, he had to show me what to do through demonstration, and there were times when he even came in while I was showering and yelled at me to do it his way. Normally he would not know, but his way of showering meant getting wet, turning off the shower, then getting soaped up. After getting soaped up, I would then rinse off the water and soap and turn off the water and towel off. My father even showed me how I should dry myself.

I guess there is something to taking a shower his way in saving water. Since I saw this method of taking a shower recommended on a show later on in my life as a means to save and conserve water. This may be so, but I still like to just leave the water running while I take a shower, and besides it is the females of the world who take the extra long showers. I have heard it told by my wife that it is because of her hair, but it doesn't make sense to take a twenty minute shower over hair. She complains that I do not take a long enough shower, and do not get clean enough.

My cousin and I had a contest once to see who could take the fastest shower. My cousin won this with taking a show in less than a minute, but I didn't think it counted because when he came out of the bathroom with a towel around his waist he was dripping wet and covered with soap suds. The funny part of this was that his mother came downstairs and saw him just as he came into the living room to have me stop timing him.

One thing I remember about my father when I was growing up was that he did not have any patience especially with his children. If something was not done his way right away you were yelled at and sometimes even got punished for not doing something the right way like handing him a tool while he worked on his cars. My father attempted to teach me how to change the oil and do routine maintenance on a car, but instead of allowing me to do some of it, I was only allowed to watch and hand him things, I do not think he trusted me in doing anything. There was a time when I was older when he allowed me to do something , but he got angry with me if it was not done right. There was no room for mistakes with my father. Unfortunately the only way to learn things is by making mistakes, this is one thing I found with my daughter who made a lot of mistakes when she was growing up, but she was determined to do things herself and her way no matter how many mistakes she did make.

Needless to say, my father had a temper and lost it easily. I inherited that temper and while growing up lost it sometimes when people were not around. There were a few times I got so angry with my older sister that I screamed at her and then got into trouble later. I also got upset with a friend who would not let me in his house so as I pounded on the screen door, I broke the glass. I also made my sisters, mother, and father mad at me as well. One time while my sister was chasing me around the house, I ran out of the house and when I hit the screen door handle to open it, the handle did not open, but my momentum carried me through the door. My arm went through the glass and cut my arm, and I nearly tore the door off.

My parents were upset with me for doing it, and got mad at my sister as well for chasing me. I think it was hard for them to get too upset with me since I was bleeding, and they were busy administering first-aid to be too upset about the situation. I think that they had me do extra chores to pay for the door. I did that a lot while I was growing up.

I broke a window when I was pounding on it to scare away a cat that was sleeping in my window well, "Meowing," all night long making it so that I could not sleep. I tried to get rid of the cat, but it didn't leave until I broke the window. Then there was a television I had to pay for at school that I was blamed for breaking, and a window at one of my friends how that I was blamed for. My parents later helped me through a church mission and college by saving up some money for me.

I do have to thank my mother for all of her patience with me and my father and being an intermediate when my father lost his anger and came after me and my sisters with a belt or started to kick us. She was the opposite of me and my father, and rarely got really mad. My father swore and cussed on a regular almost daily basis, but I only heard my mother swore once and that was when I threw up blood on the carpet after I got my wisdom teeth out. There were a few times she would chase me around the house as well and then when she would corner me, I would just hold her back while she attempted to hit me. It became a comedic routine since she really could not hurt me, and so she would just start to laugh about it and then I would laugh as well.

When I did get older, I was stronger than my father and he knew it, so he thought twice before he would come after me with his belt. Once I hit him in the stomach when he was hitting me and he stopped and after that never came after me again. Now this may seem to be extreme in a family and some may say even abuse. But this was just the way I grew up and it was common those days, or at least that was what I thought. My family would not deny that my father went too far sometimes. Yet we did not know what all of this meant. There were no doctors especially in mental medicine who could help at that time, and back then you just did not see a psychologist unless you were insane.

Now looking back, I can understand a little of what my father was going through, and I have had to work really hard to not go too far with my daughter and all of the things she does. It is like two people with ADHD clash especially when they have a temper and are related to each other with Scottish blood running through their veins. My daughter has a will of her own and if she doesn't get it her way, she loses her temper, and I am the same way about her if I do not get my way. I have had to use a lot of techniques to control my temper and to be mindful of my thoughts and where my emotions are heading. If I feel getting really angry and know that if it continues I will lose my temper and take it out on something or someone, I take a moment to reflect on what is happening and make a conscious effort to calm down and take a different approach with my daughter.

"My way or the highway," is a good motto that I have been living with, but it is not very effective and can be very hurtful to others and cause problems for me. I have a hard time opening up to other ideas. The first thing is that I have a hard time in groups. I seek the attention of others, and enjoy the credit for doing things in a group, but my shy nature makes it hard for me to join groups or to work cooperatively with others. I can manage okay if I am put in a group situation and I will mesh with the group when I need to. But I like to have things done my way.

When I was working on an administrative license in education, I had to be in a group for group presentations and projects. The problem was that I hated having to get together outside of class, and to wait on others to do their part in the projects. It worked out that my group was not too much into the group thing either, and allowed me to do all of the work and then they would check it and things worked out great. I felt more comfortable being able to get things done early so that I did not have to worry about it. Unfortunately I did not learn much from other members of the group and did not improve my skills in working with others in a group.

I have also run into snags working with administration as a teacher. In education there is not just one boss in a school. There is the federal government, the state government, and the school board. Then there is the superintendant, and then the school administration which makes for a lot of politics and bosses telling what should be taught in the schools. It then makes it even harder when there are teachers with ADHD and OCD who want to run their classroom a certain way. I am one of those teachers who likes to run my classroom a certain way with being able to be flexible in my lessons and have students do projects in my class. But with the way I think, it has caused me a lot of stress as well as a lot of antagonistic feelings towards those in charge of education. I would like it better if we went back to one room school houses where the teacher is in charge of everything in the school.

At home it has been hard to do things my way, because being married it is a partnership. I am a strong believer in partnerships and having an equal relationship in a marriage. But with my stubbornness and thought pattern it has been difficult sometimes to cooperate or compromise. Instead of a win win situation, it often comes down to win lose where one of us has to give up or sacrifice something we want to do. The key is to be able to be heading in the same direction with the same long term goals for the family with both husband and wife working on those goals with a single objective in mind and that is to be able to strengthen the family.

When it comes to being a father, I believe there are times I am being like my father and dictating what my daughter needs to do because it is my way or nothing. My daughter has inherited the same genetic disposition for ADHD that me and my father have along with the Scottish temper and pride which has caused my daughter and I to get into some very strong arguments. Neither of us are willing to give in. As a parent though I always have the time out and restrictions I can enforce which helps to resolve the disputes, but these punishments do not solve the problem and my daughter turns out resenting my decisions.

I am not saying all people who have ADHD have a my way attitude, but I know that with ADHD it becomes hard to focus unless it is on something that you are interested in and generally what you are interested in is part of your way of doing things which can conflict with someone else's way of doing things. As an example a boy with ADHD might like to listen to music while he works, but his teacher does not allow him to listen to music in her class and insists he give her his music player. He refuses, because his music player was given to him for Christmas and does not want to depart from it because he fears that someone will steal it. An argument erupts in the classroom and the boy is sent to the office.

The boy does not understand why he cannot listen to music while he does his work, because he does it when he is at home and it helps him concentrate on doing his work. Only the teacher is enforcing not only her rules, but the school rules as well. No matter how much the boy argues about his right to listen to music while he does his work, he will not win this situation and will end up losing his music player for a few days and get suspended for arguing with the teacher.

Is there a better way to handle the situation? The boy believes he is right and the rules are stupid. The teacher and the administration believe they are right, because music is a disturbance to the class, and besides they do not know what the boy is listening too which could be music with mature lyrics unsuitable for school and children under the age of seventeen. The school has a no tolerance policy when it comes to electronics in the classroom. Yet this boy has a no tolerance when it comes to working with his music.

What ends up happening is the boy shuts down first in the classroom with the teacher he got into an argument with and does not do any work for his teacher because he does not like his teacher or the class and he feels he cannot do his work without his music. Then he stopped doing his work in all of his classes all together, and eventually drops out of school because they would not allow him to listen to his music while he did his work.

This seems absurd on both sides with the school not seeking out other ways to help the boy, and the boy not willing to let go of his music and seek to come up with other ways to do his work and following the school rules. Then there are the parents who are pulling out their hair trying to understand what is happening with their son and why he is not doing any of his work at school.

As an adult with ADHD it might be that a person might get into an argument with his boss over how things are run at the business and how he is doing things. The employee might have come up with a certain way of doing things in the company that works for him, but it is not company policy, so he gets reprimanded for doing something that is against company policy. Either the employee gives up doing things his way and conforms to the company standards, or he eventually is fired and must look for a job in another state.

Living with ADHD means for me that I need to step back and look at things other people's perspective and attempt to see how they look at things in order to be able to work with them and understand their positions. This has helped me tremendously in being able to work with others and being able to overcome some of my thoughts of jealousy or envy when someone takes off with an idea that I have to follow, but do not necessarily agree with.

It is also important that there are many ways of doing things to accomplish the same goal. Things can get done even when it is not done my way. I have to be humble and teachable when it comes to the things around me and being able to have friends and be respected by others. Respect is something that cannot be given to a person through education, wealth, or fear. It has to be earned through hard work and being able to work with others appreciating their contributions to projects and other things that they are able to work on.

I have been blessed with a wonderful understanding wife, and a good natured daughter who understands that I am a little stubborn sometimes. I have also been blessed with a good job with great people I work with who are able to share with me some of their ideas and expertise. One thing that I love is to be able to learn from other people, especially people who are able to amazing things and work with others in making things happen.

Again it has been hard for me in the past and even now to be able to work with others mainly because of my shy nature, but also because of my stubbornness and desire to do things my way. But I am learning that it is important to be open minded and to take a few steps back to look at a situation in order to be clear headed enough to be able to make the right decisions.

Chapter Four: Getting Help

With all such disabilities it is important to seek help from the experts those who know about ADHD and what treatments that work the best. For children the first place to seek help would be at your child's school. Teachers, counselors, and principals may know enough about ADHD to be able to refer you to district specialist and doctors who will be able to help. They can even be able to start working with your child who may be suspected having ADHD and be able to come up with a plan with accommodations that will help him to be able to pass his classes.

In children it is important to identify ADHD early enough to be able to work on effective treatments that will help them succeed in school. Many children are able to function normally in school with the proper treatment and they will be able to start to do things that will help them to be able to control their minds and become free from distraction so that they will be able to do their assignments.

Your family practitioner might be familiar enough to help to treat you or your children if she has had training and experience with it. She might be able to refer you to a specialist or another doctor who is more trained than she is on the effects of ADHD. It is important to be working with a doctor who knows about ADHD and effective treatments and is willing to help explore several different treatment methods.

It is vital that you learn as much as you can about ADHD and in turn teach your children what you have learned. By learning about ADHD you will be able to have access to greater knowledge, understanding, and freedom. There is a lot more to living with ADHD and treatment than just going to a doctor and getting a prescription to drugs.

It can be difficult at times especially as an adult to be able to go to someone who is a specialist and be able to get the help you need, especially when those who work with ADHD generally work with children and not adults. If you are not having a lot of difficulty living with ADHD you may be able to do your own research and come up with your own management plan that can work for you. When it comes to ADHD it can be expensive seeing a doctor and getting the medication to treat it, some medical insurance companies may not pay for the treatment and the medication because it is considered a mental disorder, and we have not done well in the United States in mental health and many insurance companies do not cover mental health.

You just have to weigh your options and see what works best for you. If you have a child who can see a doctor and get an effective treatment plan that your insurance will cover you can count yourself blessed. There are always alternatives and many options you can look at. You can go with your family doctor, or you may check out a child psychologist who specializes in ADHD. Since I grew up there is a lot of research out there on the symptoms and treatment. There are several new drugs they are using as well that can help children and adults with living with the disorder in order for them to be able to overcome their distractions.

It is important to look at ADHD as something that needs a complete management plan and not just the use of drugs. The drugs can be useful and very effective with many children with the symptoms, but some of them may have negative side effects like depression, and some children or adults may not respond well with the drugs. There are the standard stimulant drugs that are used in most of the children with ADHD and then there are non-stimulant drugs that they are using as well. The rule with the drugs is to try them and come up with the proper dosage. If the drug is not working then discontinue use and seek out something else that will work.

I do not personally use a drug and I do not even take pain medications. Generally medications have side effects and if they are taken on a regular basis can lead to more serious side effects over a longer period of time causing problems with kidneys, liver, and heart. So far medications used for ADHD have been proven to be safe for use, but there has not been long term research on the effects of long term exposure to the drugs. Many children will be able to grow out of ADHD and will no longer need to be medicated through their adult lives. This is hopeful for many children who have to take medicine on a regular basis for their condition. The other thing that is beneficial is that the medications if used properly are not addictive, and will not cause severe withdrawal symptoms if the drugs are discontinued.

If you have your child on a drug in treatment of ADHD and it is working then continue that treatment. You will need to make certain, however to work on a more complete method of treatment as well which includes a healthy diet, exercise, stress management plan, and a system of organization which will help them be more organized and prepared for things in their lives.

Living with ADHD means living healthy overall. It is important in a family that the person who has ADHD is treated as part of the family and not an outcaste and that the family supports them through eating healthier dinners and by exercising together. There are times when a child who is suffering from ADHD is treated as the black sheep of the family the one who is the trouble maker and causes problems for everyone else in the family. It is important that the child is treated as part of the family and that it is the family that changes routines and habits to accommodate the child.

This does not mean enabling the child by rewarding their behavior and allowing them to get away with breaking rules. There are no excuses, and ADHD is not an excuse to break rules and not attempt to do something. I do not allow my students in my class to use ADHD as an excuse for their behavior in my classroom. There are enough treatment plans to help children that they cannot use it as an excuse to behave badly or to not do the work in class.

Often when a child learns that they have ADHD they will use it as a device to manipulate their family and other people. Parents will also use it as a means to manipulate or excuse their child's behavior. I have often heard parents come in and tell me that their child has ADHD as if it gives their child a get out of trouble free card. If the child is treated special because of having ADHD, he will continue to use it as a tool to manipulate people and get what he wants including getting out of work, and using it as an excuse to break rules at home and at school.

Children like adults who have ADHD need to have set boundaries and expectations. Strict structure and discipline is essential in the success of children with the disorder. Once the children realize that they are being treated special and do not have to do the same things as other children they will let go of their management plan and allow themselves to be more distracted than before and it then becomes more difficult for them to be able to accomplish their goals.

As a parent it is important to seek help and do research as you help to develop a management plan with your child, and then stick with the plan altering it when necessary if things are not working well. Make sure that your child sticks with the plan and monitor your child's behavior and performance at school. It is okay to reward your child and to encourage your child just like you would any child.

You can think of ADHD like any other condition a child may have to monitor like any other learning disorder. It takes patience and a experimentation to see what works the best. You may also find that what worked the year before no longer works, or that you may need to change the plan according to lifestyle changes or changes in the child's life such as moving to another school. Something like a move to another school can put a lot of stress on a child and cause him to let go of his management plan.

Do not assume that your child is following her management plan, she might be following it when she is around you, and then when she is not around you she does what she wants to do. It is just like if your child was training for the Olympics. If she continues to do well with her sport then she is training right and is continuing to train, but if your ability diminishes then you know she is either not training, or she is not training right, or it could be that she needs to change her routine.

As an adult with ADHD you need to seek help as well. It can be embarrassing to go to a doctor or to admit that you may have it and need help, because it is generally seen as a childhood disorder. You might not have severe symptoms, or have to worry about it as much because you might not be in an academic setting, or your job enables you to be able to live without worrying about it as much. But if you are going back to school, it could be a challenge to be able to pass your classes, and be able to concentrate on what is being taught.

Even at work, you might be experiencing moments of lack of concentration which is essential in your job. You might be distracted when your boss is explaining important information related to your job, and because you were not paying attention you were not able to perform your duties on your job correctly. It may even be hard for you to keep a job, or maintain a healthy relationship with anything. If this is the case you need to get some help so that you will be able to have a productive life.

You may even have turned to drug addiction or living a risky lifestyle because you have an urge to satisfy your desires and seek pleasure in your life that you associate with as being happy. Only it is only temporary and once the high of a new relationship or drug wears off you then realize your mistake. This is a good indicator you need to get help to overcome not just your risky behavior, but to get your ADHD in order to be able to function properly.

Many adults need help just like children. For children it is up to their parents to get the help for them and to attempt to help their children as a family support. Adults will often deny they are having a problem or will try to result the problem themselves. It many cases this can take place, especially if the adult is able to be responsible enough to develop his own management plan and to share this with his family.

I learned through my own mistakes that it is hard to be able to do it alone. As a child I was alone simply because my parents did not know I was experiencing this and did not know what it was. Since I was passing my classes at school they thought that I did not have a learning disorder, and I thought that I was doing okay as well. It wasn't until I had to take the major standardized tests to get into college that I was having serious problems trying to get a good score on the test.

I had always been a slow reader and had a hard time comprehending what I read. Only I was able to manage to not have to read everything at school and was able to get out of having to read a lot in high school. I had to read a lot more in college, but was able to skip through the books and only review what I needed to pass the classes. My ADHD has had a huge impact on my relationships which I hadn't realized until after I had gotten married.

In the past not a lot was known about ADHD and so it was difficult for me or my parents to seek help and develop a plan. Especially when we did not know that I had it. Even today with all of the resources and research that has gone into it. Many people who suffer from it do not get the help they need, or are unable to understand what they have and be able to come up with an effective treatment plan.

After I had learned that I have ADHD, I really did not know what to do about it. I was already at a point in my life that I did not have to worry about it as much since I had my master's degree and was married. But since then I have realized that it still impacts my life and I need to follow daily routines and work on disciplining myself through exercise and diet in order to maintain a little sanity. I have done some research and have worked on my own management plan that seems to work. I have been fortunate that I have not gotten into drug addiction or have had rough relationships.

It is now my daughter that my wife and I have to worry about and come up with a plan to help her get through school and have healthy relationships. We have been working with her in school and with her relationship skills, but there are a lot of things we still need to teacher her about in order for her to be able to have success in school and in her relationships. So far we haven't had the need to seek out a medical expert, but if it gets to the point we are unable to help her we will see a professional who will be able to give us some alternatives.

Not all children have ADHD, in fact not that many do, but there are a lot of children who have similar symptoms because teenagers tend to be in a stage of their development that they explore their boundaries and do things that normally would seem to be insane. Even if your child does not have full blown ADHD, it is important to be able to come up with a management plan to help her to be able to control her emotions, have healthy relationships, and be able to be successful in school. There are a lot of other great books out there that talk about what you can do as a parent to help your child.

Think of it as if you do not work on being able to manage your child's behavior, it will be far worse later on, and it might be the school or the law enforcement agency who will have to manage your child's behavior for you. I believe that almost all children are capable of controlling their emotions and behavior if they get help from the experts and have support from their families.

The children who end up having serious problems are those who did not get the help they needed early on and those habits and life is out of control. It often takes a handful of people to be able to work out a plan for a child. At school this team can consist of the principal, a counselor, and several of the student's teachers. It may even include a district specialist who is able to give the expert advice on ADHD. If the child is on an IEP then a special education teacher may also be present. It is important to be able to have your own team to help assist the child's ADHD problem which can include parents, the child, a doctor, and the school counselor.

As an adult you may want to assemble your own team with your doctor, your family, friends, and any expert who may be able to give advice and counsel. It is also important to be able to inform those in whom you are in contact with your condition and what you are doing about it and how it may affect your job, and academic progress. Do not be embarrassed or scared to admit that you have ADHD and you need extra help in certain areas of your life. It is better to be able to take action first than to be embarrassed later for something you did as the result of your lack of attention or being distracted.

Get the help you or your child needs and start to make a management plan that will help you or your child get control of your life and be able to enjoy the same things that others are doing. You and your child can live a normal life and be able to do just about anything you want to do. It just takes help to be able to live the life you want to live.

Chapter Five: The Management Plan Electronics

Now it is time to sit down and start to make your management plan. The next several chapters will look at different aspects of controlling ADHD. These things have been studied to prove to be affective, but not one single strategy will be sufficient in order to be able to control the disorder. Each one will help in its own way to alleviate the symptoms, but it is the combination of several that is more effective.

The first is to look at electronics. In our modern world technology has been able to do amazing things, unfortunately our brains cannot adapt to all of the changes fast enough for us to be able to process all of the information and be able to slow down our brains enough for us to be able to comprehend what is happening. I am not saying that electronics is the sole cause of ADHD, but it is a leading contributor to it. I mentioned that I watched a lot of television when I was younger, and today there are more and more children addicted to video games, television, internet, and texting.

Anything that is done to extremes has negative consequences. Each year people die from drinking too much water, people may be affected because they eat too much, read too much, sleep too much, and the list goes on. The same holds true with electronics, only the negative consequence that occurs with electronics has to do with the brain. Every time you text, get on the internet, watch television, or play a video game, your brain is going a million miles per hour processing all of the information.

Your brain is stimulated which releases neurotransmitters forming new connections and releasing dopamine and other pleasure chemicals in the brain which leads to addiction. The problem is that the excitement of the brain not only can lead to an addiction, it can make it so it is difficult to calm or slow down the brain, thus making it difficult for you to be able to be able to concentrate. Many activities that involve just a couple of elements help you to be able to focus and concentrate such as reading. By reading you can stimulate your imagination which in turn can form good connections in your brain. But again even reading can be done to death causing negative consequences such as fatigue and a loss of precious time spent with the family.

There is nothing wrong with seeing movies, getting on the internet, texting, or spending any time with electronics. The problem exists with the content, and the time that is involved with the electronics. If you are spending twelve hours a day on the internet you will be experiencing negative consequences because you may not be spending time with your family, your special health starts to suffer, because you do not have time to exercise.

Electronics can be seen as the fuel that supports ADHD. So whenever you or your child is doing something with electronics it is as if he or she will become more distracted through electronic use. I know that my daughter starts to get upset and more distracted when she watches too much television or is on the internet playing games. The more time spent on electronics the more the brain is feed through this form of media to the point it becomes an addiction and more time is necessary or withdrawal symptoms start to occur. It is like feeding candy to a baby who cannot get enough.

We all need a break from electronics and allow our brains to be able to relax and calm down a bit from being over stimulated. It can be challenging in a world filled with electronics and electronics are often used as another baby sitter for children. I have to admit that it is too easy to have my child watch television to give me a break from having her bother me. Parents buy their children phones and games in order to get a little peace of mind while they are driving or doing other things, only they might find that their children might have a harder time conveying their feelings, and will have more emotional outbursts because they cannot problem solve a minor crisis in their lives. The stress level might even go up significantly because the children are not used to having to deal with stressful situations, because they are not placed into a situation where they have to think for themselves.

There is a growing concern about children growing up unable to communicate with each other because they only know how to text each other. This can be very detrimental on a developmental level for children. Children may have a hard time developing cognitive skills that will help them deal with social emotional situations in their life. Not only will children have a harder time being able to concentrate on things, they will have a harder time processing information.

It is important for parents to be able to connect emotionally with their children without the interference of electronics. Spending time as a family in front of the television or on the internet may be okay some of the time, but there needs to be time the family spends in recreation, in social situations, and doing projects together solving problems. The tendency in today's high tech world in our industrialized nations is to place a lot of focus on electronics which causes our brains and emotions to rely on electronics and when they do not perform like we expect them to perform it places a great deal of unnecessary stress in our lives.

You take an ADHD child or adult who enjoys watching television, texting, or playing video games, and suddenly they are unable to watch television because the cable went out, unable to text because the network went down, or the video game went dead. This creates a lot of stress which results in a brain meltdown, because what they want is beyond their power. The child is unable to restore the game, or bring back the network. The adult is cannot bring back the cable, he can only call the company and complain that it is out.

In many cases electronics is not concrete or tangible enough to be able to make sense of how things work, so when the electronics do not work anymore and there is a lot riding on sending the email, or texting a friend about breaking up with a boy friend it will seem like the whole world has crashed. Unlike tangible real world situations where if a tire on a bike goes flat it can be easily fixed, or instead of texting the friend she calls her up and talks with her or better yet goes to her house and talks with her face-to-face. Instead of relying on getting the news from television or the internet, you forget about the news and relax in the backyard enjoying an ice cold lemonade on a hot summer day.

Electronics stimulate other parts of the brain and form connections that will interfere with such thinking processes as logic and reasoning. It does depend on the content and the reason for using the electronics. If electronics are used at your job and you spend your time solving problems and working through solutions on a computer that can help your reasoning skills, whereas if you are just watching a mindless television show that has crude jokes on it about something that is ridiculous then you might not be using too much of your brain for reasoning.

It then depends on the context and the content of electronic use as well as the time involved. If you are spending ten or more hours a day using electronics six to seven days a week, it can be excessive and will have a profound impact on your brain as well as your social state. The time spent with electronics is the time spent away from family, friends, and some things that may be more important in your life.

Many people often say that they do not have time to exercise, to read a book, or do other wholesome activities, yet they watch three or more hours of mindless television a day, or spend the time texting, listening to music, or play games on the internet. It is time for you to refocus on spending more time doing other things like exercise which will help to calm the body and brain down and help you to be able to think better. Just think of how many people in the world live without the internet, cell phones, music players, indoor plumbing and electricity. Think of how your ancestors lived fifty, hundred, and two hundred years ago. Many of us might think that people back them must have had it hard, and you cannot imagine how they survived without cell phones. But they did survive and many of them despite their hard physical labor and lack of modern technology. Many of them were also happier and healthier than we are with the lack of all of the stress we have.

Learning about the founding fathers of our country and how they were farmers and did a variety of different things or hobbies in their lives it seems to me that they were more intelligent than we are today, Washington with his creative approach to farming, and Jefferson with his enormous library in which he donated to the Library of Congress. I am still amazed at what had accomplished in their lives.

We have all of the information of the world and history at the press of a button on our computers, yet it seems to be information overload to the point that it is impossible to comprehend everything that is out there. Children often rely on one or two sources of information and believe it to be accurate when it could be far from being completely accurate. I find it interesting that if the electronic media is not stimulating enough for children they find it boring and have a hard time using it.

In the case of doing research for a paper they first try to do it the easy way through plagiarism or are unable or unwilling to dig deep into research looking at several different sources attempting to come up with the truth. The quality of papers overall has diminished when it should be outstanding. Since the dawn of technology with the internet, children should be super humans being super smart and the ability to perform many things that I could not do when I grew up without the internet. But I find that children are less able to function than they have been in the past, in part to electronic distraction.

As an example instead of working on homework a child can text a friend, play video games, and listen to music. There are just too many distractions available and too many temptations. It is like sending an alcoholic into a liquor store to buy a bottle of water. When I take students to a computer lab to work on a research project there are several students who are distracted by getting on their email, go to a gaming site, or visit other sites that do not have anything to do with the project.

I am surprised at how hard it is for youth to memorize pieces of information. It is as if the information is separate from there way of thinking to the point they can make a reference to it, but it does not sink in enough for them to be able to remember it and make it part of their long term memory. It is difficult to remember things when the brain is being stimulated through graphic violence or music with graphic lyrics. It is also hard to connect with people socially when spending a lot of time with electronic media and not a lot of time with people.

The content of the electronic media is the most important thing to consider when being exposed to technology. If the content is pornographic or violent then it will stimulate the brain causing chemical releases that will have a person experience pleasure and make it even more inviting to continue to view or be exposed to. Thus this type of media can be very addictive and can destroy people's lives. The short term effect is simply stimulation, excitement, and pleasure, but with repeated exposure there is addiction, and a loss of empathy towards others. These things will make it so a person will lose their humanity and will lose of a lot of our prized virtues such as compassion, courage, and respect for others.

Much of the electronic media can also be mindless drivel that doesn't do anything for our well being but waste time. If you are watching something that is funny in a non-hurtful manner it can be healthy for you to laugh, and sometimes watching a program to relax and allow yourself to enjoy something that takes you away from the stress of life can also be beneficial. But to watch a reality show that exploits the absurd behavior of people who make dumb decisions could have a negative effect on how a child might perceive that this is the way people act in real life. It might be in certain parts of the country or the world, but do you want your children to grow up as these people being their role models?

We tend to act like what we are most exposed to. So if we are exposed to a lot of violence then we may have a short temper and think that acts of violence are okay, and it is okay to hurt others especially if they deserve it. If a man is exposed to pornography he may treat women with little respect and think of them more as sex objects than people. If we are exposed to a lot of reality television we might believe that we are in competition to kick our friends off the island, or out of our lives so that other friends can compete for our attention.

Yet if we are exposed to things that challenge our thinking and force us to solve problems we will be able to handle challenging situations in our future. If we are able to look at other people's perspective and show empathy to others we will be able to get along better with them. It is the Karma of technology. What you are exposed to will come back to you whether it is positive or negative.

The other element when looking at electronics is the context at which it is used. If you are using technology as part of your job then you do not have a choice, and it is part of how you make a living, but when you have free time then it should be doing something like hiking or riding a bike. I have a neighbor who is a forest ranger and he told me that on his leisure time he doesn't want to go on a hike, because that is his job and he does it all of the time. So if you are in front of a computer all day long it wouldn't make sense for you to come home and spend all of your free time in front of a computer.

There are also many uses of technology such as online or mobile banking, connecting with people you are unable to physically go and see, and being able to complete assignments for classes. All of these things in the context of the task are appropriate for the exposure of the electronics. Even using electronics as a form of entertainment is okay for a small amount of time. But to use electronics on a regular basis to engage in negative practices, or to just waste time cannot be a good thing.

I sometimes find myself on the internet first looking up something I wanted to know more about for a writing project or for teaching my class, but then I am easily sidetracked to something else and before I know it I have spent a couple of hours surfing the internet reading information about someone that I do not need to know about like a movie star. A person with ADHD the internet can be a very hard place to be since there is just so many distractions.

Just looking on a news site there are so many advertisements that it is difficult to be able to focus on just the news and not click on one of those internet advertisements about how to lose weight, or some way to save money on home costs. It can be maddening how many distractions there can be and having ADHD you just have to click on everyone in order to get all of the information.

It all comes down to being able to control electronic use with your children and with yourself. Look at the context at which it is being used with work and school taking priority and limiting use for entertainment. Monitor how much screen time is being used every day and every week. There is no fast rule about how much exposure to electronics is harmful, but you should be able to determine what is excessive and what is manageable. If you are spending more than two hours a day on the internet, or watching television it may be too much for you, plan time to do other things in your life, like stimulating your brain with active conversations with other people, or gardening. Examine the content of the electronic use, and eliminate things that may be pornography or may contain too much violence. This can be very damaging to children and can also affect adults in negative ways.

The key would be to be able to manage and control your use of electronics and not to have it control you. The first thing to do would be to look at patterns or habits of electronic use. You might find that you spend four hours watching television at night, or you text your friends all day long. Identify those areas you feel are obsessive and start to work on scaling back on these. As a parent you will want to keep track of the electronic use of your child to see when he is texting or listening to music or on the internet, and come up with a monitoring plan like having computer and television in a family area and not in his room where he can use it anytime and have access to any content.

You can have parent controls and block a lot of content, but there will still be content that will get through filters that you may deem inappropriate for your child. The idea is not to control your child, but to be able to monitor and work out a plan in which your child will be able to understand and use electronics wisely. It is not a good idea to forbid a child from using electronics, because they will be exposed to them at one point in their life and need to be able to learn how to use them appropriately and be able to manage them.

I know some parents do not have internet, or television in their home, which is fine, but their children still need to be taught about using the internet and television and some of the negatives and positives involved with such use. You do not want them learning from their friends when they go over to play with them. Children will be exposed to a lot of things during their life, and if they are taught about electronics and some of the good and bad things that come out of the technology then they will make better decisions about their electronic use. It is also important to teach them about how it affects their brain and how using too much electronics will cause their brain to be over stimulated and will result in being more distracted and having a harder time concentrating.

Even as an adult it is important to be able to learn how to use electronics appropriately and be able to understand the positives and negatives of technology. By using technology appropriately you will be able to save a lot of time and things can work out better for you at work, school, and at home. But using technology inappropriately can lead to a lot of wasted times, distractions, confusion, and problems with relationships, trouble at work, and can lead to addictions.

The rule is to live a balanced life. There is a whole world out there and it would be a shame if you spent half of it in front of a screen, or that you ended up losing your family and friends over a senseless addiction. It is not a good thing to do anything in excess, and for someone with ADHD electronics and technology can be a fine line between genius and addiction. Just remember balance in your life and be able to do a variety of things in your life that can compliment what time you spend with electronics.

For every hour you are in front of a screen you should spend exercising, or doing some recreational activity.

Chapter Six: An Active Life (Exercise)

The best by far way to help manage ADHD is through exercise. Just through spending at least thirty minutes a day doing some sort of aerobic endurance exercise like running, biking, or swimming you will feel better, have more energy, and be able to concentrate more. Thirty minutes is not a lot of time and can be very easy to incorporate into your schedule. You can start out by walking and then increase your intensity as you get into better shape. As with any exercise routine you should consult your doctor and check to see if there might be any complications to starting an exercise routine.

What does exercise do to help your ADHD? Exercise increases the efficiency of the cardiovascular system and the respiratory system in circulation of oxygen throughout the body especially to the brain. With an increase in oxygen to the brain, the brain is able to function better and you are able to think more clearly. Just think about how hard it is to think when you do not have as much oxygen to the brain because you are sick, have a hard time breathing, or have a headache because of tension and the brain is not getting enough oxygen.

It is difficult to concentrate when your brain is being starved of oxygen and thus exercise helps to provide the necessary oxygen for the brain to function properly. Exercise has so much more benefits that it would be ridiculous not to exercise. There have been several studies over the years that have proven students who exercise are able to do better in school. Exercise does make you smarter and in the case of a person with ADHD it helps to regulate their thoughts and they are able to not be as distracted.

What kind of exercise should you be engaged in to help with ADHD? The exercises you need to focus on are the ones that will help administer more oxygen to the brain which would first start out with proper breathing and then it would eventually lead to aerobic or endurance exercises that get the blood pumping to vital organs such as the brain. After you have gotten your breathing and endurance exercises down you would then need to add strength exercises in order to keep your muscles toned and functioning properly. Just like in anything in life it is important to keep your body in harmony with each of its parts, and variety is key here with being able to do a variety of exercises and activities in order to make exercise fun and exciting instead of boring following the same routine day after day.

It is important to follow a set routine with some exercises you do every day so that it becomes natural and a habit, but it is also important to mix it up a little. By doing different exercises and recreational activities it will help you to keep interested in exercise and will be able to help you change from one activity to the next building better strategies of the brain to be able to manage your thoughts.

Breathing is essential for life. You can go without most things for several days, but you cannot go for more than a few minutes without breathing. In a crisis situation it is the oxygen that is the most important. Emergency personnel first check a person's breathing and if she is not breathing they attempt to restore it through CPR. Even the compressions are used to pump the oxygen around the body and into the brain to attempt to keep the person alive and bring them out of it with an AED. Anyone with a breathing illness will have a difficult time doing a lot of things because they will lack the energy and will have a hard time with their thoughts.

If you look at infants they breathe appropriately which is known as belly breathing. In fact they got their oxygen in the womb through the umbilical cord which was attached to the belly. When the breath goes down far enough to raise and lower the belly it is filling the entire lungs with oxygen. People who hyperventilate are only filling about five or ten percent of their lungs. If you breathe to where your chest is rising, but not your belly you are not filling up your lungs. The breath must be forced down to the stomach in order to fill the lungs.

Sit up straight either in a chair or while you are sitting on the ground and place your hands clasped over your stomach over your navel or belly button. Now inhale through your nose and allow the breath to flow all the way down till your hands are raised, and then slowly exhale allowing your hands to fall. Take several slow breathes concentrating on having your hands rise and fall with each breath.

Once you are used to breathing in this way inhale for a count of three, hold the breath for a count of three, and then exhale for a count of three. Practice this several times and then return to normal breathing allowing the breath to fill the lungs and then on the exhale attempt to expel the breath longer attempting to get all of the breath out of the body. When you inhale you get the oxygen you need to survive, and when you exhale you are cleaning the body getting ride of toxins and other things you want to get out of your body for you to be healthy. One reason why people get sick is that they are not able to get rid of the toxins from their bodies. This is why people go through cleansing their bodies.

The first step in cleansing the body, however, is to be able to breathe properly and get rid of the toxins on the exhale. Our bodies recycle air several times a day, and if you are able to become proficient in breathing you will be able to manage cleansing the body from toxins that enter it on a daily basis. By breathing properly you will be able to regulate the air that comes into your body and be able to get rid of the pollution that is in your body.

One you have mastered belly breathing and are able to do it normally then you are ready for the next step in breathing and that is to breath out with a sound. This is known as Qigong an ancient form of breathing and exercises that has been performed for over two thousand years. It is the precursor to Tai Chi Chuan. Qigong develops your breathing practices into a higher form of breathing and exercising. It lays the foundation of all of the exercise you will ever do and if done properly can do amazing things.

Qigong alone will do wonders for someone with ADHD. As an example a student who struggles with his language arts class might do some Qigong exercises before class and will be able to concentrate better. Many of the exercises can be very simple, but there are others that can be very complex with a combined routine that can consist of several moves. The most basic Qigong would be to simply place your hands near your belly button and when you lift your hands to your chest you breathe in and when you lift your arms over your head you exhale while saying, "Chaw." You do this several times.

Another exercise would be to place your hand near your belling button forming cupped hands as if you were holding a ball. You extend one arm up and one arm back as you exhale and say, "Shhhh." You inhale when you bring your arms back together to form a ball. There can be several variations with this and the previous exercise, and you can access books, and videos at your local library.

Start out by doing two or three Qigong exercises then you can add several more and even incorporate a routine which consists of several movements together. Along with the breathing you should be concentrating on the breathing as well as the movements as you meditate you will be able to increase your chi and even be able to move it through your body. The chi is your energy force that helps to regulate the body's central functions. This is why Chinese medicine attempts to balance the chi in a person's body when he gets sick. It is said that when a person's chi is out of balance he gets sick, and in order to get better the balance needs to be restored through a variety of techniques such as Qigong, Tai Chi, massage, acupuncture, and herbal medications.

Place your hands together so that they are facing each other and then separate them so they are about an inch apart. You should be able to feel a warmth, this is your chi. In scientific terms the oxygen and food you eat will be converted to energy which warms the body and can be moved throughout the body. If this is in balance you are healthy, if it is not in balance you are sick. The thing you have to remember is to be able to breathe properly and meditate as you breathe and as you move slowly.

The next two things you can add to your exercise routine would be Yoga and Tai Chi. Yoga is the original martial art that predates Qigong and it is said that monks from India brought Yoga to china which was then transformed into Qigong and then later changed to Tai Chi. Much of Yoga is the same as Qigong with the exception of asanas or poses. The poses can be held for a period of time as a form of meditation and stretching. There are several poses and routines you can learn in Yoga. It is important to be able to be balanced and think of your entire body. So if a pose helps your legs, then make sure to do a pose for the arms, and the chest. If you stretch forward, then stretch backwards as well.

Yoga means harmony, and it is important to be able to develop a routine that is harmonious to your body and will work your back as well as the rest of your body. It is important to make sure that you start off with Qigong and Tai Chi performing slow rhythmic moves with focused breathing and warming up the muscles. Then you can go into the more intense stretching of Yoga. If you stretch without having your muscles warmed up you will get injured.

The myth that was going around about doing an exercise routine was that you have to stretch your muscles first so that they did not get injured. It is not the stretching necessarily, but getting your muscles warmed up so that they can move without being overextended. So make sure your muscles are warmed up first and then you can focus on stretching and going for a run or walk followed by strength exercises.

The Qigong, Tai Chi, and Yoga are the foundation for your exercise routine, and are the foundation for your health. Once in place you can then plan on what endurance activities you would like to do such as walking, running, biking, or swimming. You might even be involved in basketball, soccer, or skiing. Just not that some of these activities although fun to do, carry with it an element of risk. I know of several guys who played a friendly ball game with a few other guys and have caused serious injury to their legs.

Just like with everything in life it is important not to do things in excess. Examine your life and determine how much time you have to exercise each day. Make sure to include at least thirty minutes or more, but do not plan spending a lot of time exercising when you have work and other things you will need to do. You might want to start out with thirty minutes and then when you have gotten into a routine you can work on adding some time to your workout.

Another important thing to consider would be exercising without interruptions. You might want to go to a gym to be able to focus on your workout, and paying the money might be the motivation you need to go and exercise, or it might be that you get up thirty minutes earlier and workout when your family is still sleeping. If you can convince a member of your family or a friend to exercise with you then you will be able to motivate each other when you are working out. Just remember you need to take your exercise routines seriously and not spend the thirty minutes just talking to your friend when you should be sweating.

The best way to get into exercise would be to have fun with it and get excited about exercising. If you make it into something that is just a lot of work and you hate doing it, then you will not be doing it for very long before you give up on the idea of exercising. Make it an exciting part of your life and allow it to be a management tool to help you with your ADHD. If it is someone you care about like your children with ADHD, then make exercise a family affair, something you do as a family in the mornings or evenings as part of your daily routine.

It needs to be something your children would want to do, so make it fun. There are a few books that have been published on teaching children Tai Chi, and Yoga, and many more about exercise in general. Just ask you kids what they would like to do, and slowly introduce new exercises and new activities. The key is to be active. Many children are already active, you just have to organize some active time in their lives that is more structures so that they will be able to fall into a habit of exercising and know what forms of exercise they can do that will help them with their ADHD.

You can start out by organizing family activity nights two or three times a week playing games like basketball, soccer, or just going and swimming. Once your children are used to spending time with the family doing something active, you can then start to talk to them about exercise and how important it is for them to exercise and what it does for their bodies and minds. The next thing you can try would be to introduce Yoga and Qigong in the form of games they can be involved with.

In Yoga many of the poses had animal names like cobra, and lion. There are other poses like tree and sun salutation which is a series of poses put together in a sequence as part of a routine. You can have your kids do an animal pose and see how long they can hold the pose. The most powerful tool you can use is to demonstrate the poses through example. Your kids will naturally want to do what you are doing. They might not be able to do many of the poses correctly at first, but through practice they will be able to get the hang of it. You and your children can have a lot of fun learning Qigong and Yoga. Even Tai Chi can be a lot of fun to learn, however, it can take a while to learn all of the moves in the different forms. You can start out by breaking the forms into smaller chunks to learn and take your time to memorize the movements.

When it comes to strength exercises it is always better to start out small with little or no weight and then add weight as you go. Children especially smaller children should not be involved in lifting heavy weights. Many children are unable to know how much weight they are able to lift safely. Children see weight lifting as a curiosity, but they do not understand the mechanics of weight lifting especially how dangerous it can be if they attempt to lift weight that is too heavy for them.

I have seen a lot of children especially younger children attempt to lift weight that is much too heavy for them, because they think that they will be strong if they can lift it. They do not understand that it takes years of lifting to be strong and a lot of time lifting smaller weights before the body gets stronger. You need to teach the safety part of weight lifting first and then slowly allow your children access to lifting and resistant exercises.

The first rule would be that your muscles are warmed up. If your muscles are not warmed up then they have a better chance of tearing or getting injured. The next rule would be to go the exercise correctly, this is one reason why young children should not lift weights, because they do not lift correctly and they do not grasp the concept of the negative consequences of lifting incorrectly. They just see a dumbbell and immediately want to lift it over their heads without any concern for their back, their arms, shoulders, or the possibility that they might drop the weight on their toes. If an exercise is done incorrectly getting injured is more likely to occur.

It is better to teach children how to do push-ups, and use resistant bands than to have them use weights. When your children do get involved in weight lifting you might want to have them start out with light dumbbells, and using weight machines. Make sure to monitor your children at all times when they are in a gym or around weights. They can be just as dangerous as having children in a swimming pool. You should not leave young children in a swimming pool without supervision, and you should not leave them in a weight room without supervision as well. This is why hotels post signs near their swimming pools and fitness rooms so that they will not be liable for someone's neglect.

Make sure to plan out your exercise routines and stick with them for several weeks. You will quickly see results and you will also be able to learn what works out and what doesn't what you like to do and what your children like to do. The overriding key to success when it comes to exercise is consistency. If you get into exercise and only do it for a few weeks and then take a few weeks off, it will not be as great of an impact on your mind and body as if you continues to exercise on a regular basis.

I observed as students I coached would exercise only during the season of the sport they were involved in and then they would not exercise until the reason returned, which meant that they were only exercising three months out of the year, and they did not get any stronger or better fit than they were before. It is important to be able to exercise on a regular basis and to make it part of your life and part of your children's life. The greatest gift you can give your children would be to give them the tools to be healthy and happy.

Believe me your life will be much better if you make exercise part of your life and that of your families. Not only will it help to manage the ADHD in your life, it will give you and your family more energy with getting sick less, and bring your family closer together. There is nothing better than to be able to hike up a mountain with your family and be able to reach the top knowing that you had just climbed a mountain and to be able to look out across the valleys below and feel a sense of great accomplishment.

Through exercise ADHD can be managed better, and even if you or your child is taking medication for ADHD exercise will help to compliment the results of the medicine. For some people with ADHD they will need to take medication to help them with their symptoms, for others they will be able to manage it through exercise. But exercise alone cannot be as effective as doing several other strategies to cope with the symptoms.

I have found, however, that exercise is by far the most effective tool I have to combat the symptoms of ADHD. Even before I knew that I had it, I used exercise as a means to help me feel better, and think better. I have always been able to think more clearly and do better in school and with social relationships by exercising. When I stop exercising for a time, I can immediately start to feel the results, my thoughts are all over the place, and it becomes hard for me to think and to come up with solving problems in my life.

I become depressed and frustrated with everything. Without exercise, life becomes a miserable mess. Even just doing yoga and tai chi helps me to focus and feel much better. But I have found that I do need to do a complete total body workout including breathing exercises, massage, and meditation in order for me to reap all of the benefits of exercise.

Chapter Seven: Healthy Diet

The next critical part of controlling ADHD is to eat a healthy diet. The more research they do on ADHD the more they can see that diet has a hug influence on the management of it. Just think of all of those energy drinks out on the market and what one of those things probably does to our children. There are two things that are readily available to us on the market that have a huge influence on how we are able to think and act. They are caffeine and sugar. Both of which can be addictive. This is one reason why some food companies have added sugar and caffeine to some of their products.

With the advent of energy drinks and many people getting into green tea, caffeine is almost a regular staple in the American diet. It is a stimulant that causes the heart to beat faster and to give you a false sense of energy. The reason why I say a false sense of energy is that caffeine which is a stimulant elevates the heart rate and with this elevation gives you more energy, however, it is both an artificial way to elevate the heart rate and a temporary fix. When your heart rate has been elevated it must come down, which means there will be a crash depending on how much caffeine was taken.

The need for a caffeine fix increases in the body and you will tend to take more and more until you are taking more than what it healthy for you. The elevated heart rate from stimulants in the body starts to overwork the heart to the point that there may be serious consequences for taking caffeine. There have been studies that show that caffeine has been linked to premature babies being born, and increase in miscarriages. It can also cause problems with someone suffering from ADHD. Even though it is a stimulant like what many of the drugs used to control ADHD, it is often abused to the point that it will cause more harm than good.

It is important to limit or eliminate caffeine from your diet and that of your children as well. You will find that without caffeine you will be able to think more clearly and be able to focus better, and not have headaches as much. As for the energy drinks, they do not provide the right kind of energy you want and you will find that just through eating healthier foods you will have more energy than you can get from those energy drinks.

Sugar is a constant in our American diet. All food has some form of sugar in it. But it is the refined sugar and high fructose corn syrup that you have to watch out for. You might not be able to find too many things in your refrigerator or cupboards that doesn't have high fructose corn syrup. The food industry has decided that they would add sugar to most products and high fructose corn syrup has replaced cane sugar.

I noticed that an average can of pop had 110 calories in the 1980's and 1990's. But now the average can of pop has over 150 calories per serving. This means that with more sugar there are more calories being added to our food. The increase in sugar puts a lot of stress on the body and causes problems with the brain. People weigh more now than in the past, and the rate of diabetes and heart disease continues to increase because of eating more sugar. The sugar does several things that are negative.

The first thing that sugar does is to increase the heart rate and increase your energy level. But this is only temporary, and there is an inevitable crash from the energy and a feeling of emptiness, thus we eat more food to give ourselves energy and fill our stomachs. We end up eating more food causing us to gain weight and be more susceptible to diabetes and heart disease. It also becomes more difficult to exercise and be active.

We often joke around about giving children something that contains a lot of sugar and say they will be hyperactive. This is in part true that sugar can give children more energy on the onset and it might make them a little hyperactive. But it will also cause them to be more distractive and have a harder time to be able to concentrate and focus on the time that is needed. Children whose diet consists of a lot of sugar will have a hard time being able to focus on tasks and be able to complete school work.

As a parent it would be important to monitor the diet of your child and to learn about what he is eating at school and when he is with friends. I have seen a lot of students coming to school with energy drinks and I am not sure if they got them from their parents or if they bought them on their way to school. Many of the energy drinks not only have caffeine they have high amounts of high fructose corn syrup as well. They are time bombs ready to go off at any time. Energy drinks are nothing more than liquid speed and should be avoided.

I have read where one person claims that being a vegetarian helped him to control his ADHD, and where another claims that eating a lot of protein will help to control ADHD. It might just be that you find out what works for you. I know that when it comes to food it is important not to go to excess either way. It is important to have protein in your diet, and even if you have made a commitment to be a vegetarian you still need to eat protein such as beans, nuts, and a combination of foods such as beans and rice, or squash and corn in order to get complete amino acids your body needs.

There are key amino acids that your body needs in order to function properly and if you are not getting these amino acids it can affect your thought process and concentration. But this does not mean that you will be able to get the amino acids you need by just eating a lot of hamburger. Some means provide little in the way of amino acid absorption into the body, so it is important that when you are eating meats that you try to eat high quality lean meats which are healthier for you.

It is also important to include omega 3 and 6 fatty acids into your diet. They help with overall health including helping the brain function properly. You can take supplements, but the best way would be to eat foods that contain these fatty acids such as fish, eggs, flax seeds, and a variety of other foods that may have some fatty acid. I like to put flax and chia seeds on my cereal and in my recopies. I also try to eat fish when I can.

Eating a balance diet is key to success with most of your calories coming from whole grains such as brown and wild rice, whole wheat pasta, cereals, and bread, as well as other grains like oats, rye, quiona, and millet. The whole grains will provide you with the energy you need throughout the day and will also help with including bran in your diet which is essential in cleaning the digestive system. Your diet needs to contain more grains that the other foods because it sets the foundation for the energy you need throughout the day. Marathon runners eat a lot of carbs before a race and the carbs they load up on are whole grains like pasta.

Be careful not to confuse whole grains with starchy foods like potatoes, and refined bleached flour and white rice. Eating too much of the refined stuff is just as bad as eating too much high fructose corn syrup. When people say you should not eat a lot of carbohydrates and they are talking about the refined stuff that is not healthy and can lead to obesity. You also need to be careful when people might advise you to go on a low carb diet. If you do not eat enough whole grains, fruits, and vegetables which are considered carbohydrate foods, you will miss a lot of the essential nutrients your body needs.

In order to eat a balanced diet and to be able to have your brain functioning at the highest level you need to be able to eat a nutrient dense diet which means one that has a lot of vitamins and minerals. The best nutrient rich foods with vitamins, minerals, and antioxidants are fruits and vegetables. Most people do not have any problem eating fruits because they are sweet. Some of the best fruits are those that are the darkest like blueberries. Many of the berries like blueberries contain high amounts of antioxidants that help to prevent diseases and higher amounts of vitamins and minerals. But just like all foods, do not go crazy with fruits and eat too many. It is best to eat fruits fresh, because the moment they are processed into something else they lose their nutrients and are not as healthy. Also when fruits are processed sugar and preservatives are added to them, making them not as healthy.

Watch out for fruit juices, because some juices will not contain very much juice, and what you are drinking is just a lot of sugar and water. Make sure that the juice you buy says it's 100 percent juice, and look at the ingredients, because many of the juices even being 100 percent juice will mostly contain apple juice which is better than a drink with just sugar, but if you are looking to buy cranberry juice because you have heard of its ability to help with urinary track infections it will not do you any good to buy a cranberry juice that only contains 5 percent cranberry juice and 95 percent apple juice.

I like to be able to grow my own fruit and eat it in season. There is nothing better than to be able to go out in the backyard and pick some blueberries and put them in my cereal, or to be able to pick peaches, pears, or apples from the tree and eat them that day. I also like to be able to pick fresh vegetables to eat such as cherry tomatoes to put in my salad. There is nothing like fresh vegetables from your own garden.

When you buy fruit and vegetables form the supermarket they are already very old and have made a long journey to the store. This means that they are not as healthy to eat, because they had to go through such a journey exposing them to the elements. Many of the fruits and vegetables can also be bought out of season because of the nature of where the fruits and vegetables where bought from.

If you do not grow your own fruits and vegetables the next best thing would be to go to a local farmer's market or farm where they sale what they grow. You will have to keep an eye out for what comes into season and when to buy. If you like to make your own juice and preserve things this would be your best bet to buy a lot of something like strawberries in season at the farm and then make your own strawberry jam that you can enjoy for the coming year.

Buying organic foods is important as well, however, there is not a big selection of organic produce and it is generally more expensive. Most fruits and vegetables are sprayed with pesticides and have been genetically altered to be bigger and look better for the public. The carrots I grow in my garden are not the best looking, but they taste a lot better and are healthier than their genetically altered friends in the produce department at my local grocery store.

It can be a struggle to get children to eat their vegetables. You should not force your children to eat foods they do not want to eat, but introduce food to them and eventually they will try it and might even like it. I thought it was strange that my daughter loved vegetables when she was two years old, but when she was six she only would eat certain ones, and this would change every month or so. One month she liked carrots, the next it was peas. She never could make up her mind as to what she really liked.

You can just make sure that there are vegetables with almost every meal and that it is presented in a way that your children may like. Even as adults it can be hard to get into eating vegetables. Try making different types of salads, and soups that contain vegetables so that you do not get bored with the same presentation of vegetables every time you eat. You may also want to try different vegetables that you have not eaten before. I decided to try bok choy and love it. It is has a clean refreshing taste to it and is very healthy. I like to cut it up and have it with my salad.

Another key to having a balanced diet is to make a lot of your own meals. For some it might be difficult if you lead a busy life, but it is worth it if you can spare the time and effort in preparing your own meals and meals for your family. The key to this is that you have control as to what is in the meal and you know what is in it and how healthy it is. You also have control over how it is prepared. For instance baking is healthier than frying, and using olive oil instead of butter can also be a healthy practice.

You might not be a very good cook at first, but through practice and following recipes you will be able to get better, and through time be able to prepare healthy meals for you and your family. You can also be able to monitor how much food you prepare. If you prepare a lot of food and are not willing to eat leftovers you and your family may tend to eat too much and it is important to prepare the right amount of food in order to eat only the calories you need for the day.

The process of gardening and preparing your own meals will help you to be able to focus better and help control your ADHD, because it give you a hobby that you can invest in and there is nothing better than working in the outdoors and reaping your harvest. Plus you get exercise that you can use. When you prepare and clean up the meals you eat it will help with your digestion and help you to be more conscious of what you are eating.

I used to make a lot of cookies and eat a lot of cookies. But looking at all of the fat and sugar that is added to cookies made me realize just how unhealthy they were. It actually gave me an idea to come up with a perfect cookie, one that is healthy. I experimented for several years and came up with a completely healthy oatmeal cookie that replaces butter with applesauce, eggs with an egg replacer, and sugar with agave. I also have included wheat germ, chia, and flax seed. I do not have a set recipe for it, but know just the right amount of ingredients to put into a bowl to mix up for my perfect cookies. They were so nutritious that I would make them for work and eat them for lunch and an afternoon snack.

A major point about diet is the amount of calories you eat each day. The amount of calories eaten each day can have a huge influence on how your brain functions. If you get too few calories you will be irritated and have a hard time thinking straight, but the same is true if you eat too much. By flooding the body with sugar it puts the body into overtime with digestion and insulin regulation and there is not enough energy to go into having your brain work properly. Just try to do your homework after you have eaten a really big meal, or attempt to be able to perform a mental or physical task after a large meal.

You should not starve yourself when it comes to your diet. But it is far better if you are on a low calories diet than if you are loading up on the calories every day. You need to figure out how many calories you need each day with how much exercise you do and your base metabolism rate so that you can eat just the right amount of calories each day. If you are consistently eating too many calories then it will be more difficult for you to be able to think properly.

I practice eating several small meals a day. I will eat meals that contain less than 500 calories so that my body will be able to process the food I eat and I will be able to use the calories I need for the day. But if I eat more than 500 calories I find that my body has a hard time using the calories and it works on trying to get rid of the calories or storing them.

Looking at animals you can see this, animals that eat less are more active and healthy than those that eat more food. Some animals will even die if they eat too much food. Just think about when feeding the fish in the fish tank. It only takes a small pinch of fish food to feed them, and if you dumb more food in the tank they will eat the food until they end up dying. Some other animals will do the same. In the United States thousands of people each year are eating themselves to death. It takes a person more time to die from eating too much than animals who over eat, but in the mean time these people are suffering diabetes, heart disease, cancer, arthritis, and many other ailments that are associated with eating too much food.

Water is another part of your diet you need to pay attention to. Our bodies are mostly made up of water, and just about every function in our bodies requires water. It is recommended that we drink 8 glasses of water each day. I find it hard to drink that much water, but I try to drink as much as I can. I can tell when I do not have enough water, when I start to have a headache and it becomes difficult for me to think right. If I drink too much water, I find myself bloated like I have just drank a lake and have to go to the bathroom every fifteen minutes.

One way to tell if you are drinking enough water is if your urine is clear when you go to the bathroom. You will also feel good when you have drank enough water. It is important that you are eating a well balanced diet along with drinking plenty of water, or you will also get sick if you are just drinking water, because it will deplete the salts, vitamins, and minerals in your body. This can be a life threatening condition which can lead to death. Every year there are people who die in places like the Grand Canyon for drinking too much water and not replacing the salts in their body.

A great deal of eating a healthy diet is to be aware of how you feel after you eat something and how you feel with the amount of water you drink each day. It is a matter of trial an error and experimentation. You just have to try out things as you try to come up with a diet that you can live with and feel comfortable with. There are a lot of factors that play in diet such as any conditions you may have such as food allergies and diabetes. It would be important to consult your doctor and a dietician if you drastically alter your diet in any way.

One aspect of ADHD is a tendency to have an addictive personality. This is critical when it comes to diet and controlling addictions. You should avoid such addictive substances as nicotine found in tobacco products, alcohol, caffeine, and avoid eating too many sweets. It is very easy to fall into consuming these substances in excess because of how the ADHD mind works and how it thrives on stimulus and seeking pleasure. This is why eating the right foods and exercise will help to regulate the chemicals in the brain in such a way that it will help the person with ADHD feel good about themselves.

I fortunately never got involved with drugs or alcohol, but I have gotten to the point where I will binge or eat too much snacks and ice cream at night especially when I am stressed out over something. I never realized that I might have an addictive personality or even knew that such thing existed until I heard a recovering alcoholic talk about it and how she said that she could not even take any over the counter medications, because she would abuse them.

After hearing about addictive personalities, I realized I was a lot like that where I needed my mind to be stimulated. When my mind was not stimulated I became bored and depressed. It was the eating the ice cream or binging that helped me feel better, unfortunately it lead to me gaining a lot of weight, and my only savior was exercise. I still struggle with eating too much sometimes, but with knowing what I have, I can control it better. In the past I thought it was just a matter of will power and self control. But there is a lot more to it that I had to look at which is more of an overall plan.

Just like with a difficulty of concentration and awareness ADHD can cause other symptoms that can be just as devastating such as an addictive personality. Through proper diet you will be able to start having a better control over the addictive tendencies and work toward a more complete plan in battling ADHD.

Weight management would be another factor in your diet. If you are eating a well balances nutritious diet you should not have to worry about weight management as much, however, if you are suffering from obesity or have a hard time controlling your weight or have an eating disorder you need to get help. It is important to be under a doctor's care and supervision and to seek advice and help from a dietician. You can also do a lot of research of healthy eating and losing weight properly not going from one fade diet to the next which can be dangerous and very unhealthy to the body.

There can be nothing worse than to put a lot of stress on the body through dieting, and it will cause you to have a harder time focusing on things and make you irritated. If you are on a diet and are losing a lot of weight it means you are putting a lot of strain on the body and will place the same strain on your mind. You may find that you will have a short temper and not be fun to live with while you are on your diet. The worst part of it is that you will go through hell while you are on your diet starving yourself, and then when you are finished you will be elated for a time and then you will fall into your old habits and start to gain weight again and then the entire process will start all over again.

You need to proceed with weight loss on a gradual schedule only losing one or two pounds a week. If you are a parent and are trying to have your child lose weight, you need to establish an atmosphere of trust and healthy eating, not restricting or forbidding eating things which will just push your child away to eat at friend's houses. It is a process that will help you to be able to relate to your child and they will be more willing to follow the healthy eating and start to lose weight the right way.

It is all a matter of working and supporting each other as well as making sure to eat healthier and focus more on the outer reaches of society and the world with all of the other children and people of the world who are starving to death because lack of food in their countries. We face a crisis of having too much whereas other countries face the crisis of not having enough. By giving of your time and money to others as well as food donations you and your child will be able to feel good inside that you are doing your part in helping others.

Thinking about others will help you to eat healthier and to create an atmosphere in your home that will aid in a better way of thinking and awareness. With exercise and diet adjusted to your lifestyle and learning what works and doesn't work in helping you to feel better and focus more you will be able to change your life for the better.

Chapter Eight: Mindfulness and Meditation

Once you have a routine for maintaining a healthy body, you need to start to work on the mind. There has been a lot of research on the mind and how it works, especially when it comes to those with ADHD. The brain is a complex organ in the body and does a lot of things to regulate the body and help use to function properly. There is still a lot that is unknown and will continue to be a mystery to scientists. Ironically the more that is learned of the brain the more they discover that the ancient practices of monks in Asia were corrects and that meditation and mindfulness seems to have the most widespread influences on a healthy mind. Once this is understood is becomes common sense that meditation and mindfulness has a profound influence on the brain and how it works.

When I was growing up there was not a lot of emphasis on meditation or mindfulness in the west. It was still just a eastern idea that was not widely accepted by the west. Since then there has been a lot of studies that have been done that proves that these things help to keep people's minds healthy. These practices are also very simple to do and do not require you to buy anything or join a club or religion.

I remember trying to teach meditation to my students and many of them thought it was weird almost like I was teaching some sort of cult. Meditation and mindfulness are more widely accepted as legitimate treatments to help brain functioning. But there was a time when you mentioned these things and people looked at you like you were from another planet or that you were part of a strange religion. It is a simple process of training the way the brain things and reacts to situations.

Those with ADHD will benefit from learning how to meditate and to have mindfulness in their lives. The brain is constantly forming and creating new connections when it is active. This is why athletes are able to get better at sports because the brain is making more connections through practice. There are amazing things athletes can do, because of the brain and how it makes all of these connections which in turn connect with the body and helps it to perform the complete movements without error.

The same goes to meditation and mindfulness where the brain will form connections and even alter its chemistry to the point that a person can change their attitude and demeanor for the better. The myths are that adults or older people cannot change, this is a false assumption, because they have found that people in their later years are still able to learn things and make new connections in their brains.

The brain can also make new connections that will go around damaged tissue in the brain to allow people who lost their ability to speak, read, write, and even eat by themselves to be able to relearn those things and have a full recovery from the accident or stroke they had. So if the brain is capable of repairing itself from a stroke or an accident, then it can overcome ADHD. Especially for children who start to use a complete plan in dealing with the disorder they will be able to help the brain to mature and make the right connections in order to be able to overcome the effects of ADHD.

When I first started to look into meditation, I had been studying martial arts. At first it seemed hard to understand how to meditate and to get the benefits from it. There were several times when I would get to the point I could master it then to lose it again when my life got busy and I stopped meditating. I had learned that it is important to be consistence just like exercise and meditated on a daily basis. It is one of those things that is relatively easy to do, it is just a matter of doing it.

In the chapter about exercise, I introduced meditation through breathing meditation and its use in yoga, qigong, and tai chi. This would be the foundation of meditation to concentrate on your breathing as it comes in when you inhale and flows down towards your belly button, and then to feel it is exhaled. Once you are comfortable with breathing meditation your can then start to concentrate on other forms of meditation.

We all meditate throughout our daily routines with watching television, listening to music, watching a game, participating in a game, playing video games, and the list goes one with how we concentrate on a particular moment in our lives. This is one reason why ADHD has a huge impact, is because it will focus our attention away from something we wish to be able to concentrate on. With proper meditative practice it will allow you to be able to focus on things better and be able to feel so much better, because you will be able to do those things you want to do such as study for an exam or do your homework.

Meditation is often associated with our senses. There is breathing meditation which we have talked about, and then there is listening meditation where you are able to listen to music and concentrate on its sounds. It is important to find an isolated area of the house or in a park where there aren't many people. Then you need to listen to music that is calm, soft, and not very loud. Classical and new age instrumental music is good for this, as well as a rhythmic bell or singing bowl that will help you to focus on the sound. Sounds and music have power effects on the brain, and have been proven to shape its structure.

Just think of how you feel after you listen to some music, or watch a show on television or a movie at the movie theater with its high definition sound. The music and even sounds will not only influence how we react and feel, it can have a long lasting impact on the brain. It is often the sounds that will make strong impressions on the brain after a dramatic event in your life. This is also why words can also have a major influence on your brain and when people say something that can be rude or hurtful it has a long lasting effect on the brain. People end up losing it when after years of abuse they suddenly cannot take it any longer and lash out against not only those who hurt them verbally but others around them.

As a parent it is important to always have encouraging words for your children and to avoid words that put down, or will hurt them in any way. These words can have a long lasting effect. Since words can have such a power effect on the mind there are monks and a lot of people who meditate by repeating words, sounds, or even will sing. Some of these words are mantras or a set of words that are repeated and mean a certain thing as they repeat the words. It can be sort of a prayer that is given. It can make a power effect on the brain to repeat words over and over again each day especially if the words are positive and have a strong meaning in your life.

By repeating your own mantra each day it will help you to be able to focus on its meaning and redirect your brain and thoughts. If all of the children in war torn countries were taught peaceful mantras throughout their childhood they would grow into being a peaceful people and would not take up weapons against their neighbors, but would have a forgiving spirits about them. The mantras will not only help you focus better on things in your life, they will also be able to help you reshape your thinking and understanding about life, and the world in which you live.

Sight is another powerful sense. We generally meditate when we look at things in our lives. Even if we cannot hear something we might concentrate through sight such as reading a book or signs as we drive by billboards. Along with sound, sight can have a long lasting impression on the brain and cause chemical reactions to take place in the brain. Pictures are worth a thousand words and they can help to cause an emotion. This is one reason magazine are able to sell because of the pictures they put on the front cover. One only has to watch television, or a movie to know the influence of sight in our lives.

Sight meditation is simply to look at an object and study it in your mind, concentrating on just the object and holding it in your mind. Buddhists might look at an image of the Buddha, and Hindus might look at the symbol for, "Om," which might also be chanted. There are some who will star into a flame of a candle, or look at an icon.

You just have to stare at an object and focus on it as you would your breathing and concentrate on all of the details of the object. This is why they object should have some kind of significance or important to you so that you can associate with it. But do not focus on an object that will cause you to have more thoughts and imaged come into your mind. If the object is more a distraction than something that will help you focus so that your mind is not so busy.

The purpose of meditation is to be able to control your thoughts and emotions. This comes when you are able to quiet the mind and remove all of the clutter that is going on in your brain. If you are having a hard time with meditation because you continue to have a lot of random thoughts racing through your mind, do not worry about it this is common. It takes a lot of practice to be able to calm the mind and be able to be effective in meditation. Your goal would be to calm the mind, be able to focus on one single thing, and allow all other thoughts to be able to float by as if they were on a cloud without interfering with your meditation. You are emptying your mind of all of your thoughts and striving for emptiness where you do not have thoughts or emotions that clutter the mind. It is like cleaning out a closet and then organizing it so that you can use it more efficiently.

You can also use your other senses for meditation. You can use incense or other smells to focus on. Some of the fragrances naturally calm and help to reduce stress like lavender. Your sense of smell is very powerful and will bring back memories especially if you had either a pleasant or unpleasant memory that is associated with the smell. It could be that someone you knew smelled a certain way and every time you smell it you think of that person, or that you might have gotten into a crash and the smell of the oil and gas stuck in your mind so when you smell oil and gas again the painful memories of the crash come flooding back into your mind.

Do not let the smell you choose distract you, but calm your thoughts and allow you to focus on your meditation. If you use the same smell in your meditation practice then it will help you to get into your meditation faster and deeper with each session. But do not rely on the smell to get you into a deep level of meditation. You need to be able to do this without external stimuli. Your senses can help aid you in reaching a higher level of meditation, but do not rely on them for your meditation, they are simply a tool to help in the process. The key is to be able to control your mind and thoughts and be able to meditate in many different situations without the use of external props.

Taste is another powerful source of meditation. All of us use taste every time we put something in our mouths. Infants use the sensation of having something in their mouth to calm them when they are upset, and associate it with contentment. Later once the taste buds have developed children start to explore new tastes and try new things. Many children then become a product of their environment when it comes to their taste and meditative eating.

In Europe children learn to eat slow and enjoy their meals. In some third world countries children learn that they do not have a lot of food to eat maybe only two small meals a day with no variety or variation eating the same thing day after day, week after week. In the United States children learn to eat fast, stuffing themselves at every meal making sure to eat everything on their plate. It is hard to enjoy a meal or meditate on what you are eating when you are shoving the food down your mouth and throat. Then the food industry adds a lot of salt and sugar to everything to the point that all of the natural flavors are drowned by salt and sugar. It is then hard to have a true experience with food unless you grow your own food and eat a meal from what you have picked in your garden.

Eating can be a very pleasurable experience and one that can help with mediation as well if it is done slowly and the mind is focused on the flavor of the food. This is one reason why seven course meals can be effective when it comes to a meditative experience with food. You should not, however, use meditation as an excuse to eat a lot of food. In fact eating slow and small portions is the best when it comes to eating meditation. Just think of our ancestors who had to grow, hunt, and prepare all of their meals. They were truly thankful for all of the food they got and focused on every morsel they ate.

Touch is also a very effective meditation and will help in the promotion of health through such things as massage and acupressure or acupuncture. Gently rubbing the hands and fingers or toes and feet can have great health benefits as well as promote meditation and help you to concentrate better on things. If you are attempting to focus on something you need to do such as study for an exam, or give a presentation take a few minutes and rub your hands, feet, and head. You will be amazed at how much better you will feel and you will be able to concentrate better. Massage helps to release your tension and allows your chi or energy flow better throughout your body.

There is even a practice of massaging the feet and hands called reflexology that charts the feet and hands with vital points of energy that relate to certain organs of the body. In China the and many Asian countries massage has been used for centuries as a method of treatment and prevention of disease. In the west there has been a revolution in the practice of massage and many massage schools have come into existence.

Touch or massage can focus your attention on a certain part of your body, as an example if you have a sore or strained muscle you may focus on that muscle through massage and it will get better. This has primarily been done with sore backs and feet. The focus of the massage helps improve circulation to the affected area and loosens up the muscles.

Couples can get closer through massaging each other. Not only is there the touch between each other, there is a sense of meditation with the other person which can be very intimate. Parents can bond with their children more through touch. This is generally why children are closer to their mothers, because of this touch when they were young that mothers give to their children. Even rough play among friends will help create a kinship that is closer than without the contact.

Another form of touch which was discussed earlier with exercise is that of movement. If movement is done properly you will focus on the movement of your body and muscles. Athletes are able to perform at higher levels because they are able to concentrate on their movement. It is through this higher focus that many athletes are able to do amazing things. You might even be awed or amazed by what some athletes are able to do and wonder how they do it. They simply are able to concentrate or meditate upon their performance better than other athletes. This is achieved in part through mental focus, meditation, and a lot of practice that connects the brains neurons to hardwire athletic moves.

You can practice movement meditation by walking. As you walk focus on things around you such as the trees you are walking by, the birds singing in the trees, and the smell and taste in the air. Walking not only can be a great exercise, but it can also be a great form of meditation if done properly. The main focus on your walk is to simply calm your mind, and focus on the things around you on your walk or hike. A walk to the local park a couple of blocks away from your house each day could be the very thing you need to overcome the stress in your life and be able to help control your thoughts and emotions in your mind and get you ready for what ADHD throws at you,

Mindfulness is a term that has often been used with meditation and it comes from the same source as that of Eastern philosophy and practices. Many noted people in the United States have made this term more common than it has been in the past, and it is a mainstay in Buddhist thought. It has even been used as an oddity in several movies. George Lucas was able to use the it in his Star Wars series as part of the force. Despite its mystery in the west and many people not familiar with the term, it is something that has always been part of our culture and lives.

You might recall your parents telling you that you need to think before you do something so that you do not do something stupid, or when you did something stupid they said, "You should have thought about it before you did it?"

Teachers may have said, "No think about it."

In the west the term metacognition defined as thinking about thinking. It may sound strange, but what it means is that you think about your thoughts in your mind and when it comes to education you are thinking about academic thoughts that come into your mind and about yourself and your abilities. Mindfulness takes things a bit further than metacognition and encompasses our entire thought process.

Mindfulness is simply meditation or focus on something or someone. You can be mindful of the food you are eating for dinner and make a mental note of how unhealthy it may be for you so that you will make a better selection of food when you go grocery shopping. It could be that you are mindful when you look at an object and notice something is wrong with it. As you are driving to school you might notice that another car is about to pull out in front of you so you apply your breaks and just miss them as the car takes out in front of you. You might be mindful of the sound of hummingbirds flying past you when you are out attending to your garden.

Mindfulness is a higher level of awareness that forces your mind to concentrate on the now and what is happening before you. This means that you are able to cleanse your mind of distracting thoughts and emotions that would prevent you from being able to concentrate on what you are doing. The heightened sense of awareness you have with mindfulness allows you to be able to do amazing things.

Just by practicing mindfulness will allow you to be able to control your ADHD to the point you will be able to function in most circumstances. But it does take a lot of practice and patience for it to work. You can start out with meditation and starting to focus on things around you throughout your day. Mindfulness is something that you can do throughout the day no matter what you are doing. It simply takes you to slow down and listen.

With cell phones, internet, video games, music players, and all of the other distractions of the world it isn't any wonder that we cannot practice mindfulness. Try practicing mindfulness every day with everything you do you will be able to slow down a bit, listen, and think about what is happening in the present. This means you need to let go of the past, what happened a few minutes ago is gone it is in the past, let it go and move on by being in the present. Do not worry about things that are in the future and you have no control over. The worry will prevent you from being in the present and being able to be mindful enough to do what you want to be able to do.

Each morning I exercise, and I have found that if I am mindful when I exercise I can get done quicker, have a better workout, and do not risk injury. If I am not mindful and think about other things, it takes me longer sometimes twice as long before I am finished with my workout, and I risk injury because I am not focused on doing the exercises correctly and may even drop a weight on my foot if I am too distracted by my thoughts. The same thing happens with just about everything else I do during my daily routine. If I am mindful of what I am doing, I do a better job than if I am distracted by other things.

Mindfulness not only will help improve your thoughts and help you to focus on tasks it will also help you with your relationships as well. You have probable been in a conversation with someone when you find yourself alone not being able to connect with people because your thoughts are somewhere else, or you are busy texting or doing something else. I hate it when I am talking with someone and I notice that they are texting or they are focused on something else, because they are not paying attention to me which means that they will not have heard a word I said, or only get half of what I was saying.

It takes mindfulness to be able to know what a person is thinking or feeling about something you are talking about or how what their feelings are about you. By paying attention and being an active listener to someone you are able to understand what they are attempting to tell you and even know what they are thinking and feeling through observation of their body language and facial expression. It is almost impossible to be able to know what a person is feelings if you are not looking at their eyes and their facial expression. The lack of communication or miscommunication between two people can be overcome if they were just mindful of each other's feelings.

This means to be mindful of someone else you need to show empathy and realize other perspectives of what people think of. Often people are unable to communicate with other people, because of lack of being mindful of what other people are thinking. You may have been in a situation where you were thinking of something else when someone was talking to you and you did not hear what the person was telling you. This means that you were showing disrespect and the person feels like you don't care about what they were telling you. You may not care or even like the person, but by not being mindful you get into a dangerous habit so that when someone you care about talks to you, you do not listen to them and the situation turns ugly.

The first step then would be a mindful listener or active listener taking an active role in listening to someone. You are looking at the person and not texting someone else. You are thinking about what the person is telling you and observing facial expressions and body language. You are attempting to not only listen to everything the person tells you. You are trying to understand what he is telling you and attempting to know what he is thinking and feeling as well. Think about how you feel when people are really listening to you and are excited about what you are telling them, the same is true for everyone. This is why humans are social creatures, because we need to rely upon each other for many different things including being able to communicate with each other and feel good when someone connects with you and are excited about what you told him.

If a person is not excited about what you are telling them, and even act like they do not care or want to listen to what you are saying, you feel sad inside and start to doubt your own self worth. The same thing happens when you are listening to other people. You have to be attentive and try to learn something from what the person is telling you.

It is often bias, fears, and distractions in the brain that break up the active listening. With ADHD it can become difficult and at times impossible to listen to someone, because of all of the distractions that are coming through the brain. It might look like you are listening to a friend talk to you, but in reality you are thinking about a video game you want to play, other friends you would like to hang out with, school, parents, your job, the piece of meat stuck in your back teeth. Your mind is filled with other thoughts that are commanding your attention, and on top of that you feel that this friend of yours who is talking with you is rather boring, and you normally tune her out to the point you don't remember anything she tells you.

The thing you do not realize is that she is insecure and is attempting to make friends with as many people as she knows, and you happen to be one of the only friends she has who will listen to her sob stories about how she is having a hard time in school and her parents are always fighting at home and are thinking about getting a divorce. The strange thing is that you do not know any of this, because you are busy tuning her out and giving your other thoughts more attention.

She finally picks up on several clues that you are not paying attention to her, because you look like you are not showing any empathy towards her after she is almost in tears about her troubles at home. She realizes that you do not really care about her, and so she ends the conversation and leaves feeling worse than when she approached you to talk with. She leaves more depressed than when she first came over.

Only you do not notice how she is feeling. You are just glad that she left and is no longer talking with you, because you are going to go play the video game you were thinking about earlier. Just think about the missed opportunity to help your friend, and not only that, you have missed an opportunity to recognize that she very beautiful not just on the outside, but on the inside as well, and she is a great person, if you take the time to listen to her. If you were also perceptive you would also find out that she likes you. But you will never find out all of this, because you are too busy with other friends you find a little more interesting, and you are busy with other things in your life and do not have the time to pay attention.

There are a lot of missed opportunities because of the lack of communication and no mindful listening taking place. I know from personal experience all of the times in my life, I missed several opportunities to get to know people better. Part of the problem I had was I was too scared to talk with people, but I did get into listening to people. There were several times I was able to be mindful enough of other people in order to be able to benefit from it. Even though I was not the smartest kid in school, in fact I was considered one of the lowest students in school, but I was able to listen to the teachers in class enough that I was able to understand the lesson and be able to do the work and pass the tests. It was the other classes, the ones in which I did not like the class or the teacher that I had problems with.

When my family moved to Ohio for instance, I was nervous being in a different place, and scared to death to talk with other people. It gave me a unique opportunity in the fact that I was in a new place and people did not know me, so they did not know of my abilities or lack thereof. I could have reinvented myself, and started fresh with people, and for a time I did just that and was able to make friends and do well. Except for in school, I soon found that it was harder than my other school, and in math I was failing so I did what any boy with ADHD might do, I shut down and blocked out the teacher and the class. If I would have been open, I would have realized that I could have gotten help from the teacher and by listening I could have learned more about how to do the problems.

When I tried out for football, I was good enough to be able to be on the team, but not good enough to play according to the coaches. The reality of it was that the coaches had already chosen their favorites and looked at me as not being that good. I again used my ADHD to retreat and not pursue the coaches to get noticed. If I would have been mindful enough, I would have known a little more about the coaches and what they wanted and would have been able to prove to them I was good enough to play. But I allowed my fears to distract me enough that I did not attempt to get the coaches attention.

The head football coach did, however, notice in my weight lifting class that I was the only one who was serious about the class and about weight lifting, and so he arranged it so that I started one game, only after a series of plays the defensive coach pulled me out and would not put me back into the game. It was also late in the season when the head coach started to notice me, if I was a junior, I would have been able to have made a better impression on the coach.

This is what life is all about, getting people's attention and giving our attention to other people. It is the art of socializing with others. With ADHD it can be difficult because of all of the distracters in the brain that prevent you from being able to concentrate on what a person is telling you. The only way to be able to overcome the distracters would be to allow those distracters to pass by as you give your full attention to the person who is talking with you. It will take practice and there are a lot of places in which you would be able to practice. You can even make it into a game where you try to tell what a person is thinking and feeling at any given moment, and that you can even start to predict what the person might say or do based on the information you gather through your mindful listening.

The next time you go to the store really pay attention to the people around you shopping. Every time you go to a social event pay attention to the people around you. It can be very entertaining to see how people act. You may even find that people are not so much different that you are in the way they act, and feel about things. I am amazed at how people really are a lot like me when I observe them at the grocery store. I do see other people who are more like aliens from another planet and have a completely different paradigm of living than I do, and these people are easy to read.

Take the time to be mindful and to meditate and reflect on the things around you. Once you do it will be like you are waking up for the first time into another world. It can be very difficult at first overcoming bad habits and getting used to focusing on other people. But in time you will eventually be able to master the art of conversation and socializing. Once you do this you will be able to make a huge difference in your life. I have noticed that most of my bosses or supervisors in all of the jobs I worked at may not have been good at things, but they were very skillful in talking and listening to people. It is an essential skill to rise to the top in a company.

As a parent it is important to be mindful of your children's needs and be able to comfort then when they are sad, and teach them how to be effective in the world. Extreme lack of mindfulness is neglect and can cause serious problems with the children. The family runs much more smoothly and children are happier and easier to handle when the parents are mindful of what is happening in the family.

It only takes a few extra minutes to be able to listen and connect with your child, and it will save a lot of time in the future. Instead of arguing with your child over little things, you are able to focus on teaching your child, and being able to connect with then to the point where you are learning from them and spending a good time with them enjoying every minute you spend with your family. By teaching children to be mindful you are giving them a skill that will help them with the stress in their life and be able to help them connect with other people including you.

Teaching ADHD children about mindfulness would be the single more important skill you can teach them, because it opens up their thoughts and minds to endless possibilities that they are able to have. It is simply teaching them how to focus and control their minds. It seems almost a no brainer when it comes to helping those with ADHD, yet we often ignore the obvious and go to treating children with drugs and telling them they just have to do it. But by teaching them how to be mindful we are teaching them how to be able to control their condition on their own without the aid of other people and without the aid of drugs. There may be some children that the use of drugs can be very effective and that would be the best route to travel on, but for the majority of children they just need to learn how to be able to think more mindfully.

Mindfulness is simply meditation, only it is a little more in depth. It requires a willing mind and an almost eagerness to pay attention to something. I had mentioned that I have had a hard time reading all my life, and contributed that with ADHD and the inability to concentrate to enough to be able to understand what I had read. I never thought I would be able to finish a book and remember anything about the book I had read. My mother would force me to read, but I hated it all of the way and never was able to read very well. It took me an hour to read just one page in a book. I was envious of my mother and others who could read a book in a week and be able to remember most of what they read in the books.

But I had discovered that I found some bodybuilding books that I was interested in that I was able to read from cover to cover and remember what I had read. Only it was not the same type of reading as before and I had found that the more interest in the book I was the faster I could read it and the more I got out of the book. It was my interest that got me excited about reading and countered the effects of ADHD.

As a teacher I see the same thing in my students. If they do not like something they will just say it is boring and will not even attempt to read or do other things in school and then they start to shut down. With ADHD it then becomes a matter of interest and forcing the brain to be able to be interested in a subject. Through mindfulness this is exactly what you are doing you are making the mundane exciting and being able to change something that seems boring into something that you just cannot get enough of. I have experienced the power of this in my own life and in the life of my daughter and others. Through mindfulness and becoming excited about things someone with ADHD is able to break through the barrier and learn a great deal about things.

It can be treated as a game or an adventure to be able to learn a lot of things through the books you read and to be able to listen to someone else and understand what he just told you about an upcoming exam. There are a lot of things you may be missing or your child is missing because of distraction, through practicing meditation and mindfulness there will be more clarity and focus and the distractions will no longer be a factor.

Chapter Nine: Routines

Without the routines in my life, I would be hopelessly lost in the confusion of my thoughts. My wife and I were having trouble getting my daughter to clean her room. She was six years old at the time and capable of cleaning her room by herself, but she insisted to the point of throwing a temper tantrum that she could not clean her room without help. This happened frequently, and I would continue to tell her that I was not going to help her and she could clean her room by herself.

Eventually my daughter somehow figured out why she was having such a hard time cleaning her room. She told us that she could not clean her room by herself, because she became distracted by her toys and would end up playing instead of cleaning her room. I was amazed by her insight, and recognized that she did have a problem, because it was something she feel into when she went into her room to clean it. Instead of cleaning her room she would start playing with her toys again, and would even create more of a mess. She did this around the house as well. It was something that for many parents would seem like she was just getting out of cleaning her room, but it was an actual dilemma she had to work through.

This situation is often played throughout the world where children and adults are unable to communicate with each other because of the different perspectives. As parents we just wanted our daughter to clean her room and there was nothing more simple than that because she was capable of it. We would often get out the big guns and threaten her that she would not be able to play with friends, swim, or watch television if she did not get her room cleaned. But in the mind of my daughter, she was frustrated because she became distracted by her toys and the desire to play with her toys instead of cleaning her room. This is often the case with most children they get distracted and are unable to

94

accomplish a task and as adults we have to keep reminding them over and over and over again until they do what we asked. We become frustrated and lose our temper often taking out on our children in one form or another and then they become confused because they do not know what they had done wrong.

There may not be a magic bullet or a perfect solution to the problem, it may take several different strategies to help your children accomplish simply tasks that drive you crazy like cleaning their room. It will take patience and trial and error on most situations to see what would work. One such strategy that may be effective is to establish routines for your children and as an adult with ADHD you would need to establish routines for yourself as well.

Routines are beneficial for everyone regardless if you have ADHD or not. They help to get things done, and to form healthy habits. I was not truly convinced about routines, because they seem a bit like being in boot camp in the military. But when I read about Eric Weihenmayer and how he was able to do things in his daily life, I was convinced about routines. Eric who became blind while he was a teenager was able to graduate from college, get a job as a teacher, and then climbed the tallest mountains on each of the seven continents. He contributed a lot of his success to established routines he had. Eric mentioned that he had all of his clothes organized in such a way that he was able to grab a pair of socks and put them on without trying to spend a lot of time looking for a pair of socks.

Think about how much time you spend looking for a pair of socks that match if you do not have your socks organized, now try to find your socks being blind. Now imagine being blind and not having a set routine, you would be in complete chaos trying to find things, and be on a set schedule. You would have a hard time doing much and what you did do would take you twice as much time doing it. This is the same that holds true for those with ADHD. Without routines it takes twice as long to do things and there is a lot of chaos.

Routines along with organization is by far one of the best ways to manage ADHD. It is a matter of developing healthy habits that are done everyday such as brushing your teeth and taking a shower. If you are able to do the same thing over and over again to the point it is a habit or a routine then it gives you more focus and direction in your life. If you brushed your teeth just when you felt like it or at different times every day or even skipped brushing your time throughout the week, then it would be difficult at best to make brushing your teeth effective.

If a child is attending school and doesn't have a routine when she comes home from school, then she will be at a loss for things to do, and will either do nothing and be very frustrated or will do things that she enjoys the most like video games or texting friends. But if she has a routine which involves doing her homework right when she gets home and then after doing her homework she unloads the dishwasher, and helps to prepare dinner, and then cleans her room, she is able to be focused and can accomplish the tasks she has to finish.

The structure of the routines is what gives the person with ADHD an agenda to follow, something to focus their mind on. The same holds true at school where the child needs to have a routine in order to be able to learn. Teachers need to have a set of routines to follow in order to be able to control their classrooms or the students especially those with ADHD will start to misbehave.

I know the days I do not have a routine, I am like a boat without a rudder and cannot steer. I have a hard time being able to do anything. It is only through routines I am able to focus and get things done. For year I struggled to write books, and it was not until I was able to establish a routine where I get up early in the morning exercise and then start to write and when I write I have a set of how many words I need to write before I am done with my writing or when I need to move on to the next thing on my list.

My routines start with a list of things I must accomplish in the order I need to accomplish them. I begin by thinking about what I need to do the next day and write down those things I need to do the most first and then put them in order of how they will appear in my day. I also include some of the main things that I do each day in my routine and then add those extra things that I need to do for that day such as a meeting or a family activity. By coming up with a routine, I am able to do amazing things as well as being able to do the events that come up in my schedule.

Routines are so much a part of my life, that if I am unable to follow my routine, I feel frustrated and upset. This can be hard, especially when something comes up that disrupts my routine like a family issue, or a work related event. The beautiful part of routines is that you can make them flexible to include those things that come up in your life that your did not expect. This means that you can alter your routine to fit those unexpected meetings or family emergencies and still be able to recover from the disruption of your schedule. If you are faithfully following your schedule then it will not hurt you as much if you have to eliminate some things from your schedule for the day.

As an example, I exercise every day, so it would not hurt me if I took a day off from exercise to do something else that comes up for that day. But if I do not exercise on a regular basis then missing another day only makes things worse because I cannot afford to keep missing days. The same holds true with work and school. If you never miss a day at school or work and an emergency comes up your boss or teacher will not get upset over the loss of one day, but if you have been absent or missed several days of work, one more day will be too much for your boss and teacher resulting in losing your job and failing your classes.

Routines need to be a set of things done each day that are habits. The routines need to be consistently done on a regular basis such as what you do every Sunday or Saturday and what you do during the week. Children need to know that they have to empty the trash or mow the lawn on Tuesdays and Fridays with only an occasional change in the schedule. Things have a better chance of getting done if children and adults know what the expectation is and what they need to do. Many of the successful people in the world have routines that they do on a daily basis in order to be able to accomplish the goals they have set.

With all of the electronic media, there are many forms of organized schedules and calendars you will be able to have access to in order to be able to create your routine and to follow it and see what your progress is. I personally like to hand write what I am doing for the day. There is something about paper and pen that helps me to remember things better than if I were to put in on a calendar on the web. I haven't even gotten into following day planners. My choice for an established routine is simply to write it down in a notebook breaking it up into morning, afternoon, and evening.

Routines can also help you stay healthy and fit through scheduled work out sessions, and menus for the day. I plan exercising in the morning and in the afternoon, as well as have scheduled in several meals for the day. Since many of the routines I have followed for a long time in my life, I am able to follow the routine without having to follow a written routine that I have to look at each day. Until you get to the point your routine is a habit it is important to write everything down and have it available to you as a reference throughout the day. If you would like you can program your routine into your phone, or electronic tablet that you can look at if you need to know what you need to do next in your routine.

When I exercise, I used to have a written routine that I would follow, but now I have all of it in my mind and I am able to access my memory of how I want to change my routine and looking my progress. From time to time, I might record what I am doing when I am weight lifting to indicate how much I am lifting and how many reps and sets I have done. By keeping track of my workout, I can see if I am making any progress on my strength or of how many reps and sets I am doing.

Routines work in just able all aspects of life including your diet, exercise, work, school, study at home, doing homework, chores, and many more things that we attempt to do on a regular basis. They can help to compel you to stay more focused and accomplish more things than you can do without them. When I was younger and I would wake up and do a lot of things in the morning. I would often think that I did more things in the morning than many people did during the week, because I was able to organize a lot of things to do in the morning, and with waking up early I was able do a lot of work.

It is hard to see other people I know who do not follow routines, they just wake up when they want to and go to bed when they want to. They are late to almost everything, and do not seem to follow any sense of patterns, and it is hard for them to be able to accomplish much. These people are the ones who sacrifice exercise, good eating habits, and time spent with family and friends because they do not have time for these things because of their lack of routines they find only the time to go to work, school, and do those things that are a must do or they get into trouble.

My daughter falls into the category of must do, and not enough time for anything else. She is still learning about routines and when she is able to follow one she is more content and is able to accomplish a great deal of things. She loves to write out a set of things she has to do the next day and faithfully follows the list until she has done everything on the list. This gives her a sense of entitlement and she is able to focus a little better than if she had no schedule. When my wife and I just tell my daughter to clean her room, she is distracted by her toys, but if she has cleaning her room on her list, she cleans her room in order to cross it off on the list. Eventually when she is able to get into a routine she will be able to do many things without my wife and I telling her to do it. Just like when we taught her to brush her teeth, and make her bed. They are habits that are part of her routine both in the morning and at night that they are to work on.

Established routines are an essential part of any person with ADHD treatment. I cannot picture what my life would be like without routines. I am not as rigid as some people are when it comes to routines, but I work hard at maintaining routines in my life. I wake up at 3:00 do tai chi and yoga, go for a run, bike ride, and weight lift. I make a cup of herbal tea and write and edit for two hours, and then I get ready for work. I always arrive at work early so that I can prepare my lessons and the things I need to do for the day. When school starts I am ready to begin my day teaching and working with students.

The lesson plans are routines in themselves. I start off with a bell quiz for the students with my essential question for the day's lesson, and from there I give a short lecture which involves instruction as well as demonstration and then I assign students an activity to do by themselves or get students into groups where they work on an activity together in their groups. Students do better in a class that is well structured and there are routines in place. If the class is chaotic without structure or routines the students start to feel frustrated and lost.

When school is over my routines continue where I go home check in with my wife and daughter to see how they are doing and if there is anything I can help them with. I then get busy with emptying the garbage, mowing the lawns, doing an afternoon exercise routine, and fixing dinner. One night a week I volunteer as a scout leader and teach the boys various skills. Even during scouts we have a routine we follow each week where we recite the scout oath and law. Another night a week generally on Mondays my family and I have family night which we call family home evening. During family home evening we attempt to have a routine where we say a prayer, read scriptures, and give a spiritual lesson. There are times we will go out and do something fun like going to an arcade, or go on a hike. We might even make cookies or brownies. We will even play board games together.

Just before bed we have a routine of saying prayer, reading scriptures, brushing teeth, and reading a book. When all goes well we follow the routine and get to bed at a decent time, but when all does not go well and we do not follow the routine things do not go so well. Our daughter does better when we have routines for her to follow. If we do not follow a routine, then she starts to act up and it becomes a fight to get her to go to bed and settle down. A big part of the disruption of not following routines is watching television. We will get watching a movie or one of our favorite shows and it will get late and we will forgo the routine with the intent to just go to bed, only our daughter is then wound up and unable to just go to bed.

The hard part is also when there is a break in routines with vacations, holidays, weekends, birthdays, and all of the other special occasions that come up. It is hard because we will be moving forward with everything going well with our routines and then we go on vacation or have a family get together and the routines are broken and it takes us a few days to get back into the routine, and in the mean time we are all going through stress. It is as if for a time we surrender to ADHD and allow it to rule our lives causing a lot of stress and frustration. In the mean time we are rationalizing in the back of our mind that we just need a vacation from our routines and everything will be okay. Yet we are running around not knowing what to do and wasting all of this time.

Routines need to be consistent meaning that you do not take time off on the weekend, throw out the routines in the summer, or decide that you need a break from routines for a while. It can be as disastrous as giving an alcoholic the freedom to take a few drinks now and then, and providing him with the alcohol. Leaving routines will only result into falling into bad habits, and if you have had a lot of bad habits before you had gotten into routines, it will be easy to fall back into those habits and get caught up in them like an addiction.

You may think that this idea of having routines in such a strict way is kind of like the military and can be a little obsessive to the point that it could be unhealthy. Yes that can be the case if you become obsessive to the point that instead of routines helping you have control of your life that the routines control your life instead and prevents you from doing some things that you would prefer to do. The routines can be bad if they provoke any negatives in your life.

Routines need to be consistent and done on a daily basis and not broken very often in order to be more effective and be able to control the effects of ADHD. Routines also need to be flexible and you should be able to change them when you need to. Life is full of changes such as moving to a new house, changing schools, getting new friends, getting a new job, and changing your goals and interests. Thus you're routines out of necessity will change, and the nature of weekends, summers, and special occasions will be cause for change as well. You will have a different routine for Saturday and Sunday then you will during the week. When your child wants to play soccer and they have to go to practice three times a week you will have to change your routine.

I idea is that life is full of changes and things happening all of the time. It doesn't mean that you abandon your routines, but alter them to fit your life, and you maintain routines in order to keep a little sanity in your life. Without the routines then you will find yourself rushing to places and trying to pick up all of the pieces of your life. It can be more challenging and more difficult to be able to accomplish your goals and get things done without routines and without a sense of order in your life and that of your children who will be wondering what to do without an agenda or routine to follow.

Another vital part of routines would be able to reflect on the effectiveness of the routine and come up with ways to improve it and make it better. Take the time to evaluate your routines and go over any changes you need to make and how they will fit in your life. Once you have established the routines in your life they will become automatic to the point that they are as simple as brushing your teeth every night before you go to bed. The routines will just become part of your life and you will not worry about them and they will become part of the background of your life.

Chapter Ten: Living with ADHD

Living with ADHD can be a nightmare for both a child and the parents. It can also be a nightmare for adults who have ADHD. There are varying degrees as to how it affects people's lives. It can be as simple as just having a hard time concentrating on some things such as reading or listening to someone tell you something. But it can be as severe as causing depression, and an inability to function in society to where a person cannot pass classes at school or keep a job. This could lead to drug addiction, mental illness, and a host of other conditions.

The treatments and understanding of ADHD is far better than it has been in the past, however, the early detection and the process in which people get help still needs a lot of work. Many people especially adults will go years with ADHD not knowing they have it and believing that they are just stupid and do not know how to learn. Children may suffer for years in school trying to get good grades, but not knowing that they could do a lot better if they were able to control their distractions. Many children may believe that those distractions are normal and everyone goes through the same distractions.

You may not really know if you have ADHD and do not want to have to go to a doctor and go through all of the long process of evaluation and spend a lot of money just to find out you or your child doesn't have ADHD. If you or your child is easily distracted and is having a hard time reading, or doing well in school no matter how much she tries. You can start to treat her as if she has ADHD and make sure she is exercising, eating a healthy diet, and getting organized through routines. You can also practice mindfulness and meditation in order to be able to have control of thoughts and stress. These things are just good for all people regardless of if they have ADHD or not. It will not hurt you to get started on a plan now and you should be able to see some amazing results.

The only element that diagnosis and medical treatment offers is the use of the drugs that treat ADHD. Doctors may also give advice and counseling to help with the treatment process. This may be the course of action that you may choose to follow and it may be the right choice. The use of drugs can be very effective in helping to treat the symptoms of ADHD and allow children to live a more normal life.

Living with ADHD, however, means more than just taking drugs. It means changing your lifestyle such as eating healthier, exercise, being mindful, practicing meditation on a daily basis, and follow a set of routines in your life that will help you stay organized and focused. You can get help from those around you as well as professional help, but ultimately you will have to do a lot of this alone and know that you will have to drive yourself to accomplish your goals and follow your routines.

I know that for me living with ADHD has been a monumental struggle of trying to do well in school, being a good kid at home, and trying to accomplish some of my goals in life. There were several times when I just wanted to give up on life and take my chances in the next one. Fortunately the Lord has seen fit to keep me here for some reason. Maybe it's to help people who struggle with ADHD in their lives.

I was fortunate to survive high school and get my diploma and go on to college and even getting a master's degree. I do not know if I will go after a doctorate degree, but I do know that I am now an avid reader and love to learn new things. Not long ago I decided that I would learn more about fly fishing. I had only done it once and did not know much about it. So I bought a fly rod and checked out a lot of books from the library and even bought a book. I read up on fly fishing and since then have practiced a little, but I am still not very skilled at it. Maybe when I am retired and have a lot of free time on my hands, I will get more into fly fishing than I am right now.

As an adult with ADHD, I have struggled through college, and getting a job. I am able to do well at the jobs I have had because of my drive to do my best at the jobs that I have had, yet I found it difficult to remain at some of the jobs and be content with them, because of getting bored with the jobs and always seeking something better, something that paid more money or challenged me more. I ended up having several jobs until I finally got a job as a teacher.

Teaching is challenging enough and can be just the right job for me, because it changes and I am able to change how I instruct the students and it gives me an excuse to learn more about things in the world. I started out my teaching career teaching geography and I have found out that geography is perfect for someone with ADHD, because it is so broad and diverse in nature. I could talk about the other countries of the world and examine both the history and the current events of a country as well as all of the rich cultures the world has to offer.

It is like how if you eat the same food day after day you will get bored with what you are having and you will not have any enthusiasm for dinner. But if you spice up your meals and change them on a regular basis you become excited about eating dinner and enjoy all of the variety of meals you can eat. This is what geography is to me, it provides the variety and diversity that I so crave to keep me from getting to bored. It also gives me the excuse to be part of the different cultures that I learn about and experience them.

I might not be able to travel the world, but I am able to experience a little bit of Europe, Africa, and Asia through learning about them and learning about their cultures. Not only can I see the different places with

Google Earth, I can listen to the music that might be played in a village in Pakistan or eat the same type of food that is served in a Brazilian café. Living with ADHD is all about being able to not only overcome distraction, but to be able to fill your thoughts and mind with enough excitement to hold your attention for a given period of time. For me geography does this as well as learning about a lot of other things that can help me to be able to be excited about life and excited about what I do.

Live with ADHD is different for everyone, some people have a lot of support at home and school and it doesn't affect them as much and they are able to have a very effective treatment plan that works for them. But there are others who do not have the support of family and friends and are unable to get the help they need from a medical professional with having access to the drugs, and they fall into depression and drug addiction living from day to day seeking the next fix that will help them feel good for a time and then they will crash and wish that they were never born.

I found it difficult living with ADHD mainly because I did not know what I was dealing with and thought when I was younger that I was just more stupid than the rest of the kids at my school. It was hard for me to read books and not know what I was reading and to reread pages over and over again not knowing what I had read because my mind was not paying attention when I read the page. It was frustrating to take a half an hour to read just one page and then not knowing what I just read. I honestly thought that I was just stupid, and that it was amazing that other students were able to read a page in only a few minutes and my mom who was an avid reader could read an entire book in only a few days.

I thought that students who did well in school were superhuman in their abilities to remember what the teacher said and to be able to do the assignments and get A's in the subject. For the longest time I thought that I was an outcast, that at the least I was adopted from some strange part of the world where people were not able to do things like they did here. I even allowed my imagination go and thought of me being from another planet where the people might not be able to read like they do here on the Earth, but that they had other amazing abilities that I did not know yet I possessed.

But as my life went on I realized that I was trapped in this nightmare and I was not going to wake up in a world where I was like everyone else and I was able to read and do well in school. The problem was, I did not know what was going on with me and I did not take the time to pay attention to other students and realize that I was not the only one who was struggling and there were other students who were going through the same thing I was going through. I was not alone, only I did not know this, because I was caught up in my own self pity and did not recognize that I was not a freak and there were other children who had ADHD along with me and who struggled with reading, as well as other things at school.

On top of all of this I was extremely shy and terrified to talk to others and seek help from the teachers. I also lived at a time that children where best to be quiet and not ask questions. Students who were noisy at school were severely punished, and I would also get punished at home if I asked for help. I was to be quiet, and if I was quiet then I was not yelled at by an adult, so I went through my life not asking for help and not questioning to find the answers to my life's questions.

Another thing I experienced living with ADHD was that of my father living with ADHD. I had thought of my father when I was growing up as being mean and harsh at times. He did go too far at times when it came to discipline and there was some verbal abuse taking place with me and my sisters, but given the times it was somewhat common for adults to be this way among children. It was not till later that I had learned that my kind gentle grandfather had been harsh with my father at times as well.

One thing that added to the mix of parenting was that my father was characteristic ADHD. He was often very active and unlike me talked a lot. I imagine him in school acting a lot like some of the students I have who are very hyperactive and talk a lot. I am not sure if my father got into trouble a lot at school. He probably feared what they would do to him if he misbehaved because when my father went to school a teacher could give their student the strap, and then the kid got the strap when he got home as well. It was a double dose of corporal punishment.

My father also had a lot of outlets for his ADHD which many kids chose not to do. He would run around with friends down near a river and through what today would be considered a forest. My father also rode horses and when he got old enough went to work. He worked when he was a teenager all the way through to retirement without a break.

When I was growing up, I did not know much about my father's background. It was not until much later some of the things he had experienced and some of the things he had to deal with. He had gotten married young and quickly had three sons he needed to raise. Then he went through a divorce, and ended up meeting my mother. With my mother my father had four children three daughters and myself. I had two older sisters and one younger sister. M

I remember me and my father going fishing and doing some things together when I was really young, but this stopped when I got into sports and was a little older. It seamed that my father and I were somewhat close when I was young and then we went further apart. I started to resent my father, he did not take me fishing one summer when he had promised he would if I did not play football that year. He also started to turn mean and verbally abuse me calling be stupid and getting upset with me over really small things like spilling a glass of water or trying to ask him if I could get something to drink before bed. It was as if he was my enemy.

I hated myself because I did not please my father, and I hated my father because he did not treat me well. I attempted to run away from home once and became chronically depressed. It seemed like I was in a dark deep pit and there was not one who was willing to lower a rope down to me.

It was not until later on when I was an adult that I had learned that my father went through a lot of stressful situations when I was young. He had lost his job as a parts manager for a store and he struggled for a time to find a good job, then he also went to college and worked to get his degree. Plus he had the stress of raising four children. Then there was a time when he hit his head while he was working at home and started to have seizures, and had to take medication for it. On top of all of this he also had ADHD.

The thing about ADHD is that the brain is not a patient brain and it demands action and stimulus. I found out the hard way that my father was not a very patient man and he lost his temper a lot. The added stress of work, school, and raising a family along with ADHD was just too much for my father at times and he would lose his temper and unfortunately for us kids we were the ones that were often the ones in the line of fire when he lost his temper.

I am convinced that my father did all that he thought he could do given the circumstances to raise a family and do the best he could as a father, husband, and do his job well. He provided for his family financially and was able to raise several children all of which turned out good. Now if he was able to know that he had ADHD and would have been able to have done something for it, he would have done better in life, and would not have taken it out on us kids.

He would have also have treated me differently if he would have known that I had ADHD. It would have still been a struggle for my father and I, but at least we would have understood each other better. It wasn't until I was an adult and I realized that I had ADHD and my father had it as well that my father and I have gotten a lot closer and I have realized all of the things he has done for me and my sisters. We cannot change the past, it is done and over with. I hold no grudge to my father for what he has done in the past. I have moved forward and my father has moved forward. It is what happens in the present that matters the most, and hopefully we both will help each other out.

It is also the next generation that I am concerned with now. Since I have been involved with education and learned more about ADHD, I know that my daughter is just like me. She can be very hyperactive when given the chance, and extremely shy when she is placed into an unfamiliar situation. She had driven me insane at times and has been out of control. Yet with knowing what she is going through because it was what I have gone through and knowing that she is having a difficult time in her life dealing with the constant distraction, I am not only able to help her, I am able to relate to her condition.

There have been times that I have lost my temper and times that I have overreacted to situations, but I have been able to quickly recognize my error and work to overcome it and resolve the problem. I have had to learn more patience in my life and work harder than I have ever worked in order to teach my daughter about how to behave and do her school work and other things in her life.

One thing I have learned from my experience growing up has been to praise my daughter when I can and to show to her that she is capable of amazing things in her life and she is not limited or an outcast like I thought I was when I was young. My wife and I are able to nurture and help her with her talents and help her overcome her

111

weaknesses and make them strengths. My daughter doesn't fully understand what is happening with her, but she is starting to figure it out and do something about it.

We are enjoying life more and having a lot of joy in our life knowing that we have something that we can control and even help us to fulfill our goals in life. I know there is no cure for ADHD. It is a condition that is more of a challenge or obstacle that is placed in our path that we have to find out a way to get past it and overcome it and move forward with our lives. My father had never gone to a doctor to treat his ADHD, and I have not gone to a doctor. Maybe we should have gone to a doctor in order to have overcome what we both have. I also have not taken my daughter to the doctor as well. Many because it has not affected her school work as of yet, and doctor's can be very expensive, this is one reason my father and myself have not gone to see a doctor.

I am not saying that you should not seek medical attention, it may be the best option for you to choose for yourself or your child. But for some of us that is not really an option. Therefore we have to life with ADHD and do the best we can to overcome the symptoms and work hard at doing the things I need to do.

Just like living with any chronic illness like MS, or diabetes you need to know everything you can about the disease, and then come up with a management plan that you will be able to do for the rest of your life and stick with it making some necessary changes along the way. It takes a lot of hard work, patience and a determination to want to be in control of one's brain and thoughts in order to accomplish the things I need to do. Just like in the management of MS or diabetes you will have to have set routines and control your diet, get out and exercise, and then practice meditation and mindfulness in order to develop a sense of awareness.

The key to living with ADHD is not to let it control your life, but to be able to control it and use it to accomplish your goals. Through controlling your ADHD you will be able to be in charge and be able to do the things you so desire to do without having to worry about not being able to accomplish it because you have ADHD and become distracted all of the time when it comes to working on your goals. This means that when you sit down to study or read a book you are able to do a variety of techniques to help you to remember the materials and be able to do well in the class.

For instance, In order to be able to pass my classes. I paid a little closer attention to what the teacher said in the class and I then would skim through the text to find the things I felt were important information the instructor had mentioned and then wrote down some notes to help me remember what I wrote down. I ended up passing my classes and in many instances even got an A or B out of the class. The same thing happened when I went to write a paper. I would go through the research and write down the reference as well as some notes about what I had read, then I put it together in a logical sequence and then wrote my paper based on my notes. It worked out so well that I was able to do very well on my papers. Everything I have done I have had to come up with a system in order to be able to accomplish the tasks at hand. When I am at work and am given a task to do, I come up with a system to get it done.

I like to make lists. Before going shopping, I make a list of the things I need to buy so that I am not tempted to buy a lot of things I don't need. It also saves me a lot of time just wondering around the store. There are lists for things I need to buy, lists for things I need to do each day, lists of things I need to finish for the month, and lists of goals I would like to accomplish. I have filled up a lot of notebooks with lists of goals and things to get. Even though I may not refer to those lists after I have made them, they help me to process some of the things in my life that I need to do or would like to accomplish. The lists help to organize my thoughts and my life a little better than if I did not make the lists.

My management plan in dealing with my ADHD is not completely sound, but it does help me to lead a more normal life and I have been able to accomplish several things over the years such as completing my college education, and getting my black belt in TKD. The plan I follow is simple, I exercise, try to eat right (This is my weakest area), have set routines that I follow religiously, use mindfulness and meditation to help calm my thoughts, make lists and organize things in my life, and follow a set of core values that I believe in and are important to my family.

Chapter Eleven: Core Values

No matter if you have ADHD or not it is important to be grounded with a set of core values you live by. These values help to set a foundation for you to be about to follow and practice in your life. The values are what ground us to our beliefs and what we feel the strongest about and have a major commitment. The most successful people of the world will follow core values and it is the core values they practice that helps them to be successful and not just by earning a lot of money, but by giving to other people through charity and helping their community.

Core values are what people believe and live buy, it is what motivates them to do things on a long term basis and motivates them to help others and strive to do better with their lives. When a person does not live up to their core values they become depressed and frustrated with themselves and life. It is as Shakespeare put it, "To thine own self be true." You need to be true to your set of core values. If you decide to go against your core values you will be miserable and lost and not know what to do with your life, and if you decide to go down a path that takes you from your core set of values then you will be in trouble along the way.

In order to follow your core values you need to understand them not just buy what they are, but the meaning behind the label on the value. Another term that may describe our core values would be virtue. Our values and virtues go hand in hand when it comes to looking at things in life. By aligning up our values we will be able to have something we can focus on in our lives and thus be able to revert to when our ADHD is starting to take over our lives and we are starting to lose control. We can fall back on our values and things can come back together.

You need to examine what you believe in. It might be part of a religion you belong to, or it could be a set of ethics that you follow at your job. It can also be a set of universal virtues or values that most people follow in their lives. Core values is not a set of commandments to follow or government laws to follow, they are what we believe in the most that helps ourselves as well as our fellow mankind and communities that continue to be part of society.

When I went through school, I knew that it was important to show up to school and be to my classes on time and to do my best to pass my classes and to be respectful to my teacher. I followed a set of values that were in place in my life that was part of my life at school. I really did not have to think about it, but follow it. By following these values I had for school, I was able to focus on them and not be distracted by my ADHD. So I was on time and to school with nearly perfect attendance passing my classes. There were times I had struggled to do well in individual classes, but by following my core values, I was able to easily apply myself to school and saw the need for me to follow those values.

Belonging to the Church of Jesus Christ of Latter-day Saints, I don't drink alcohol, use tobacco products, and avoid caffeinated drinks. I also don't shop on Sunday, and perform several hours of church service a week. These values help me to avoid things that are harmful to me and helps me to focus on others who need my help. I cannot imagine how my life would be without my faith and these values. I know that people who do not have this struggle a lot with temptations that I do not have and I am able to overcome my ADHD because I know that if I follow these values my life will be so much better than if I did not follow them.

Through my church, I have had an opportunity to take part in the scouting program which is based on a set of core values with the Scout Oath, Scout Law, outdoor code, slogan, and motto. These set of values which for each scout needs to be memorized helped me to focus on them when I am having a hard time in my life being focused. I know that the scouting program has been able to help countless boys to grow into productive adults in society. The Scouting program encourages service which helps young men to recognize how service helps those in their community and with their eagle project they are able to make a difference in their neighborhood.

My family is also a big part of my life and I have a strong set of values in relation to my family. I believe in keeping my family together, being kind, gentle, patient, and understanding to every member of my family. Service within the family is very important to my values, I want to help my wife and daughter and my sisters and father in anything they need my help with. Time spent with family is also very important such as having dinner together, family night, and activities throughout the week. It is important for me to support my daughter in the different activities she does, and to be able to help teach her what she needs to know like the values I live by.

I also live by a set of ethics at work which helps me to know what I am expected to do at work. This means showing up on time, working hard, and not doing anything at work that my break those ethics like lying or stealing things. Another ethical practice would not to hurt others I work with and since I am a teacher it would be not to hurt the children. It would be unethical for me to show at a child or harm the child in any way. I have heard teachers who have belittled students in their class calling them stupid or lazy, which is going against the code I live by and one at which all teachers are suppose to follow.

The strange thing about values is that they do not really get us in trouble if we break them, but that they do cause a lot of further challenges in our lives. If I am late to work, I could be written up for it, and if I did it several other times I could be fired. If I swear at a student I could also be written up and eventually fired. But there are many others things I could do that would be unethical that I could get away with and several teachers have done this. It doesn't mean that it is right for teachers or employees to be unethical and by being unethical they lose focus and direction in their life. With ADHD losing one's sense of purpose can be devastating.

It can be easy for parents to neglect their children, treat their family poorly, and do things that would not show very much compassion towards others. The core values are again not to be seen as a set of rules, laws, or commandments, but beliefs to follow and live in order to be focused and have direction in your life. Those who do not follow these core values will not have anything to be grounded to and will be lost.

I have seen this among several of my students, they start to follow the wrong crowd and their set of values are gone and they no longer focus on the good in life and the positive thoughts. There are students who sit and do nothing in my classes. I seek to give them help, but they refuse, and refuse to take part in the class. I can see it in their eyes that they have given up on life and have nothing to fall back on or to follow in their life they are completely lost. A student who has ADHD will focus on what makes them feel good no matter how negative it might be, just so long as it gets them to a level of pleasure they are satisfied with. This means that these kids get into drugs, gangs, sex, and electronics to the point that these things consume their lives, and they dig themselves into a bottomless pit they will not be able to get out of.

Students who are grounded to a set of core values they follow are more focused and work harder to pace classes and do after school activities. They have a positive path they are following and they are able to do well in school even if they have ADHD or other learning disabilities. It is amazing to see some of these children who struggle to pass math class or get an A out of their language arts class. Even though they might be distracted at time in their classes and have a hard time reading they know that they really want to pass their classes and do well in school, so they make the extra effort to do this, and in some cases it requires a lot of effort and willpower to do this.

Focusing on core values is like being able to have a major goal or something to shoot for in life despite having a challenging wall in front of you which is ADHD. I hate it when parents or students talk to me and use ADHD as an excuse that their behavior was caused by ADHD. This may be in part true, but to use it as an excuse in many instances gives them a license to lay down and do nothing. But I know better, and I know that everyone who has ADHD if they try hard enough can overcome its effects on their lives. They can also develop a plan to control it which may or may not include prescription medication and the advice of a doctor.

I am now going to attempt to discuss some core values, these by no means are the only core values, and as you might know your values may be different for the different areas of your life. You will have a different set of core values for your family then at school or work. This doesn't mean that some of those values don't cross over to other areas of your life. The core values in which I will discuss may be core values for all walks of life and situations.

Honesty is the most basic of core values. It starts with being honest to yourself and if you are honest with yourself you will be able to be honest with others. You need to do what you tell other people you would do. If you told your teacher you would hand in an assignment the next day, you need to turn in that assignment or you will be considered dishonest. Honesty is a universal core value that will impact all parts of our life. When dealing with ADHD you need to be honest about when it is hurting you, and be honest about developing a management plan and knowing when you need help.

Charity is when you do things for other people. You can look at it as performing acts of kindness, or service to others who need. You can do acts of kindness for your family, friends, people at work or school. Buy having charity in your life you are showing that you love others, and this is very important in your life and can be a very powerful motivator to do things. You can get involved in your community as well to help others in service.

Courage is an important value that will help you to do things that you may not normally do or are afraid of doing. Do not limit your life because you lack the courage to do them. Seize the moment to do your best and make your mark. Take the first step in doing things and give it a try, if you do not try things you cannot ever find out if you could have done it or not. I have seen a lot of people who have lacked the courage to do things and because of this they have lose out on some special opportunities in their lives. I know there have been several times when I have lost opportunities do have done things, but I also know that there have been several moments I have had the courage to do things as well. It was through courage I was able to ask my wife out on a date before we really knew each other, and it was courage that helped me get through college, get a masters degree, and to take the plunge and write books.

Those who have ADHD must have courage to be able to meet the challenges in their lives and to be able to overcome their learning disability in order to be able to accomplish their goals. It takes courage to admit that there is something wrong with you and to seek help for it. It also takes courage to face your fears and to overcome them.

Self-discipline is also another very important value to work on, because it is an essential part of overcoming ADHD. Self-discipline is what helps a person to be able to have control in their life this is why exercise, proper diet, and routines are important because they help to develop self discipline which brings control in your life. It not just involves discipline of the body, but it involves discipline of the mind as well. A big part of having ADHD is that your mind is racing with thoughts and emotions that come across the stage of your mind, and through self-discipline you will be able to control those thoughts and emotions to the point that you will be able to entertain only those thoughts that are of benefit to you and others and then dismiss all others that are negative in nature.

Disciplining the mind is part of the mindfulness and meditation that was spoken of earlier in the book. Through meditation and being mindful of the thoughts in your mind you will be able to take charge of your mind and develop a disciplined mind that will help you to be able to focus on the important things in life, like being able to do well in school, at work, and in your home with your family.

You need to be able to value responsibility. The greater the responsibility the more you have to be able to fulfill that responsibility. The higher you go at a job the more responsibility you will receive, and the older you get when you are a kid the more responsibility comes your way from your parents. Responsibility can be exciting and scary at the same time, because it could mean that you are in charge of a car when you receive your driver's license, you may have to pay insurance and bills. You may be responsible for employees or children.

The things you are responsible for will determine what will happen in the future. If you prove that you are dependable and can handle the responsibility then more responsibility will be given to you. If you just got your driver's license and your parents allow you to drive and things turn out okay, then they may give you a car that you will be responsible for and soon they will have you drive your brothers and sisters around for them. You will also be able to drive around with your friends and go places that you want to go to because you have proven that you are responsible and dependable.

This is all what friendship is all about being responsible and dependable when challenges come up. At your job you will move up and your boss will really like that you are responsible. At school you will find that a lot of opportunities will open up to you in whatever you get involved with such as sports, being a student body officer, or just doing well in your classes. It might be hard to focus on things with ADHD, but if you remind yourself of your responsibilities it can help you to focus a little better.

Another key value is to be respectful. Respect is frequently talked about, but often misunderstood. Gang members see respect as having people fear you because you have a reputation for being a good fighter, and being mean to others. Respect is the opposite, it is where you do something because you care about the other person, not because you fear them, or that you know that you know you will get into trouble if you do not do what they want you to do or tell you to do.

I had a lot of respect for my parents and so I did not get into trouble at school, because I knew that it would hurt my parents. I respected my master when I was taught taekwondo through bowing and doing what he asked me, because I cared about him and admired what he was doing. So this means that for respect you need to obey your parents, teachers, and those around you not out of fear or because they want you to, but because you want to. Even though my ADHD caused me troubles at school, I worked hard to get good grades out of respect for my parents. In part because I knew I would get into trouble, but mainly because I knew it would hurt them to know I did poorly in school.

The greatest reward from showing true respect is that it is a reflection back on you. Through showing respect to my parents, I was able to do better in school and other areas of my life and I felt like I needed to do my best not for myself, but for others. In other words the person you show respect for will often have great concern and caring for you, and will want you to do things that are in your best interest, thus helping you to get where you want to go.

Living with ADHD you need to rely on your values to help you focus on the most important things in your life. You need to ask yourself what is the most important things that you value in your life. For most of us it is our family whether it is with your parents, our brothers and sisters, or with our wife and children. You may also value friendships and the people you work with. By keeping your values in your life, you will have the courage to do new things without thinking that you will not be able to do it because you have ADHD. You will be able to respect others and have charity to seek to help those you care about as well as those you do not know.

Life is a grand exciting place to be if you are focused on your values and are true to yourself as you seek a place to belong in this world. You need to start with your values and they will lead you on the right path to take. If you do not follow your values then you will take the incorrect path in life and become the vary person you do not want to be. ADHD will not have power over you and you will be able to concentrate on the things that matter the most in your life.

Chapter Twelve: The Outdoors

In the book, *The last Child in the Woods,* it talks
about how children have a deficit of nature in their lives,
and mentions that one reason why children have ADHD is
that they spend a lot of screen time in front of a computer
or television and not enough time outside exploring. I can
relate to the book and it holds true to what is happening
with the coming generations of children. Instead of the
outdoors being this exciting wonderful place to be, it is
becoming less available to children.

Sure there will be backyards and playgrounds, but
this is not the same as spending evenings and Saturdays
exploring fields where there are rabbit holes, lizards, and
beat up club houses that you are your friends built to have a
place away from home to meet and talk about life's most
important things like girls, school, and going camping.
There is something in all of us that compels us to go
outside to listen to the birds singing, sit on a porch swing to
feel the evening breeze as it flows through our hair.

Even those people you spend most of their time in
an office, at home in front of the television and hate the
idea of camping and sleeping on the ground, will admit that
there is something to going to places like the Grand
Canyon, and Yellowstone that is just simply amazing.
These places call out to us to go there and to see the glory
of God's creations. There are millions of people who visit
the National Park Service parks every year, there are even
millions more who venture into BLM and National Forest
lands.

Yet many children would prefer to be in front of a
screen then to go out and play or go on a hike. It isn't that
they don't really hate it or even understand what it means
to go on a hike, and if they were to just try it they might
even like it. I know that I have taken students of mine on

hikes and virtually everyone of them love the experience and wonder why they hadn't done it before.

So what does the outdoors have to do with ADHD, and how does going on a hike help a person with ADHD? It has to do with the senses. In the outdoors there are so many opportunities to explore your senses. It is like going into a jungle gym of senses. There are a host of smells, sights, sounds, tastes, and things to touch that it gives the person an opportunity to meditate and contemplate nature. Despite all of the stimulus for the senses, it also allows people to calm the mind and be able to focus on each of the senses separately and all at the same time. One moment you will be listening to the birds sing and the squirrels chatter, the next you are smelling the pine and the wild flowers as they come into bloom.

The outdoors is the perfect classroom for the ADHD student to be able to allow their minds to explore, be creative, and just let go. It is amazing to see children who are normally off the wall suddenly calm down and enjoy being out in nature. There is something about nature that resets and recharges the mind. The more time a child can spend in nature, and the less time in front of an electronic screen the better.

I noticed early on with my daughter that when she was outside she was the happiest and was able to deal better with her emotions than when she was inside most of the time. She would scream as loud as she could when she was a baby, but when I would take her outside on the deck to see the backyard it would calm her down and most importantly it helped calm me down as well. We would feel the cool breeze on our faces and watch as birds flew over and the trees swayed with the wind. I was not sure why this happened, but I knew there was some magical powers at work when my daughter was able to go outside and in particular when we would go on hikes together she loved them and it stimulated her mind to the point that she would excitedly talk to me when we went on hikes and talk about what she was seeing and hearing along the way. It was as if she was a different child when she went on the hike.

I had loved the outdoors when I was growing up as well, only I was not fortunate enough to go camping as often as I would have liked. My parents were not avid campers, so I do not remember too many times we went camping, and when we did go out it was to drive though Yellowstone or some national park. My grandparents and cousins would go on trips and I would join them, but the older I got the less I went out into the wilderness, despite the fact that every day I went outside and could look up at the mountains and they were only minutes away.

There are a lot of opportunities to be able to get outside and explore the many millions of acres of nature. The learning and adventures are endless when it comes to the wilderness areas of the United States and Canada. There is just so many things you can do in the wilderness areas near your home that you can spend a lifetime exploring and learning about everything within sight of your house.

It wasn't until I was in my 30's that I realized just how important nature was in my life. I had signed up for a three week course in the wilderness to explore the mountains of Wyoming. It was something that I had wanted to do earlier in my life, but I didn't have the money and doubted that my parents would have allowed me to go on such a trip. Ironically my father drove me to the place where I was to start my trip and picked me up. During those three weeks, I felt more alive than I had ever experienced in my entire life. It was not easy and there were times when I felt that I might not even survive the trip, and I longed to be back home eating pizza in front of the television. But it was an experience that I will never forget and not only was the experience amazing, I was able to meet other people in whom I was able to grow close to over the course of the class.

Since that trip, I have been able to go on a couple other trips one in Yellowstone where we spent three days backpacking along the Yellowstone river. I went on a couple of solo trips where I spent several nights camping along and hiking through the mountains. It gave me time to reflect on my life and think about all the things that were happening. Then I also have gone on several hikes in the mountains not far from my home. I had never made the connection between my involvement with nature and how it was affecting my life until later, but I find that the time I spend in nature helps me to stay grounded and focused on life and gives me a better perspective of how I should live my life.

The lessons, I have learned while in the outdoors far out way all of the lessons I have learned in school and in college. Just three weeks in the wilderness was like spending an entire year in a college classroom. Many of the lessons in nature have a direct impact on life itself and especially when it comes to ADHD.

Tom Brown known for his tracking skills and the outdoor survival school he founded in New Jersey taught in his books how to be aware in nature and to be able to learn everything about nature. Through his long comprehensive study of tracks with the guidance of an Apache scout he was able to know the true nature of what was around him. He had developed a sense of awareness that allowed him to be able to track animals and people through just about any terrain and to discern what was happening to them. Through his outdoor classes he has taught thousands of others the ways of the woods that he has learned for himself.

I have not yet taken one of his classes, but have read all of his books, which are amazing. Through reading his books and spending time out in the wilderness, I have been able to gain greater awareness of the woods that I have traveled in and with life in general overcoming my ADHD tendencies. The best way to describe this experience is that when I go on a hike or camp it is as if I am traveling to a different world one that is free from the technology and the fast pace life that most of us follow.

The solo trips I have done in the wilderness have brought a whole new understanding to life for me. They were able to help me open up my mind in a way I never thought possible. I was able to have a clear almost empty mind that allowed me to speak to my very soul. It was as if for the first time in my life I was able to see myself for who I really was and to spend some time with myself and look at myself as if I was out of my body observing what I did and getting to know me from the perspective of an outsider. It amazed me at how vivid my thoughts and all of my senses were to the point that it scared me.

I went to the Henry Mountains which is in the southern part of Utah south of Hanksville near Capitol Reef National Park. The Henry Mountains are on BLM land and are isolated from the rest of the state being a small mountain range consisting of a few peaks of which Mt. Helen is the tallest at over 10,000 feet tall. The Henry Mountains also sit on the Colorado Plateau which makes it at a higher elevation. At the base of the mountains sits a desert landscape that does not receive very much moisture during the year and is a stark contrast to the mountains as you climb in elevation.

I went there to be able to prove to myself that I could do a solo backpacking trip and to have some time away from my family. I also had hoped to see some American Bison since the Henry Mountains are home to a herd of buffalo. But driving up to the mountains and hiking along the road up the mountain, I was not able to see any buffalo. I did see a lot of buffalo chips, and some evidence that they were on the mountain. When I drove up to the mountain there was not another sole that was there. I parked and camped just into the mountains with the intent of leaving my car and hiking up the mountain in the morning.

In the morning I went up along the dirt road that led to a campground that looked abandoned because there were no people there and it looked like there hadn't been anyone there for quite some time. I noticed a small stream running through the campground one of the only streams I would see on the trip. I had brought a lot of water to sustain me on my trip, since I had read that the Henry Mountains did not have a lot of sources of water.

My journey on the lonely dirt road led me up to a flat area on the top part of the mountain. It was a night area and I had decided to camp there. The isolation and solitude of the mountains was pleasing and terrifying to me. I liked being alone, and yet I was scared being alone as well, not that I was scared that I was going to be attacked by a wild beast or some people, but that I was scared being alone with myself and listening to my own thoughts.

Part of the reason why I had done a solo trip was that of self discovery and learning more about who I was, and this was the perfect place to do this, only it made me scared to find out who I really was. My entire life I was told by others that I was worthless, and I had to some extent believed this. Being alone on the top of the mountain I was able to face those fears and to think about who I really was and if I was worthless. Another part of me also wanted to get closer to God, and to have my own personal revelation as to who I was, what God thought of me, and if there was a purpose for me in this world.

It is like going on a vision quest. I had read about Native American beliefs and practices and the one thing that appealed to me the most was the vision quest and to know more about how to get my own vision. I guess I was scared that on the top of the mountain, I would learn the truth that I was a failure and that everything in life was just a joke and there was nothing special about me and about my life and when I died there would be no one to morn me because I had not done anything great and people did not really know me and those who did know me didn't think I was a great man.

Part of these fears did come to me while I was alone. There were a few other people who came up on the mountain in trucks, one group that consisted of a family was even going to camp just below where I was camping, only when they heard me making noise above them in the woods they ended up moving on. For some reason I became scared of the people who came to the mountain not out of fear that they would be able to hurt me in any way, but fear that they were intruding on my personal vision quest and that I would not be able to receive what I wanted to get from the trip.

During the night the wind blew loud battering my small one man tent making it difficult for me to fall asleep. It sounded as if a storm was approaching and I fully expected to have gotten rained on during the night, so it surprised me when I got up to go to the bathroom, that the sky was perfectly clear of clouds. I sat back on the top of the mountain on a ridge and looked up at the sky and billions of stars shown back at me as if I was floating in outer space. It was the most spectacular site I had ever experienced at night looking up at the stars. For one of the first times in my life I realized how insignificant Earth really was and that there are millions of worlds out there with intelligent life and of those people they were millions who were contemplating the same things I was and may be looking at the sky like I was wondering what was out there and what it all meant.

At that moment, I was not worried about my ADHD or anything else in my life or in the world. I was just in awe by it all. It was only the chill of the air that forced me to go back to my sleeping bag in my tent and to attempt to get a little sleep before I woke up. I had brought notebooks and paper with me to attempt to write while I was communing with nature, only my thoughts were not on writing. I did write some words in my journal about the experiences I was having, only I could not think of anything else to write about. I was not able to be inspired to write the great American novel or even just a good short story.

The next morning I got up and hiked up to the top of Mt. Helen where I was able to see miles in every direction and was amazed to see the desert below me. I could see all of the slot canyons to the west and the mountains near Moab to the east. After spending a short time at the top of the mountain, I went down to where my camp and backpack were waiting for me. When I reached my backpack, my intention was to spend another night there, only I had realized how much I missed my family and longed to be with them.

I did something that I really didn't think I could do, and that was that after hiking to the top of Mt. Helen, I hiked all the way back to my car and drove all the way home and still got home by late afternoon, the entire time just thinking about being with my family. When I did get home I was excited to see my wife and children again and it seemed that they were excited to see me as well. I had a greater appreciation for my family, who I was, and my life than I had before.

The next year I ventured to the Uintah Mountains on a solo trip where I intended on climbing the tallest mountain in Utah Kings Peak. After spending a week at Woodbadge training for scouts, I went to the trailhead for Kings Peak and went a few hundred yards and found a place to set up my tent. For some odd reason I really missed the people I had spend a week with at my Woodbadge training and could not get them out of my mind. The experience of Woodbadge was still fresh in my mind.

Scouting had been part of my life for some time and so when I was called to be an assistant scout master, I took the plunge in taking a Woodbadge class, which was amazing and I was able to learn a lot in the week that I was there. It was hard for me to focus on my solo trip, especially with all of the people on the trail. Unlike the Henry Mountains there were several people who went on the trail to go to Kings Peak. I ran into a dozen or more backpackers some who were just there to fish and enjoy the area, while others were there to conquer the mountain and climb the tallest mountain in Utah.

The next day I went as far as I could along the trail and decided to camp not too far from Kings Peak so that I would not have far to go the next morning to the peak. I was exhausted from the hike and after I pitched my tent took a long afternoon nap. I woke up and ate some things and wrote in my journal and read a book I had brought with me, but I was not very active and did not venture out of my tent, and it did rain on my tent for several hours in the afternoon, and wondered if it would be raining in the morning when I made my attempt on the summit.

In the morning, the sky was clear and Kings Peak was in the distance calling me onward to climb it, only I was still tired and missed my family terribly. I was still fearful of my own thoughts and being away from my family. I decided to give up on my attempt at the summit and to hike out and go home. Only after reaching my car and driving for a short distance I decided to stay at a hotel where I could get cleaned up and have a good night's sleep before going home the next day. This proved to be nice, only I resorted to my former habits of watching television. I am amazed at how many distractions there are and the temptations to be distracted so that we do not have to listen to our own thoughts as if we are terrified of them and that they will tell us the truth about who we are and where we need to go.

The wilderness is one of the only places we can get away from the distractions and be able to be with our own thoughts and to be able to think clearly and learn about our true self. You can still go into the woods and go on a hike to seek out those places in your life that help you to be alone with your thoughts and how you perceive the world in which we live in. I know that I will continue to go into the wilderness and experience nature at her finest only I do not know if I will be able to do another solo trip, perhaps in the future when my daughter is out of the house, I will again set out to climb mountains and be with my own thoughts.

Many people especially in the United States drown out their thoughts with noise. They might listen to music, watch television, play video games, listen to the radio, talk with family and friends, or text, but there is always some form of distraction that is occupying their minds to the point they cannot listen to their inner voice the one that is who they really are. It is hard to be in a place where it is totally silent to the point that there is absolute silence. I have only experienced this about three times in my life. Even when I wake up at 3:00 there is crickets making their music, trains in the distance bowing their horns, dogs barking, and as I write this the fan on the laptop is blowing, the sounds of my fingers tapping on the keyboard, and the sounds of my chair moving comes to my ears.

I remember three such places I was able to experience total silence. One was in a cemetery in Fredonia Arizona which is in northern Arizona near Kanab Utah. It is a very small town which doesn't have any stores, I believe there is one restaurant in the town and that is it. They even put a dummy in the police car on the main street so that they do not have to hire a police officer and pay him to enforce the law.

In the cemetery, I had jogged to it in the morning and went there to look at the unique head stones that are often found in small cemeteries in small towns. When I was there I stopped running and walked. I then stopped and for about two minutes there was no sound not even the sound of my breathing or beating heart. It was so odd not to hear anything that I froze and savored the experience like it was a precious moment in my life worth all the gold in the world. I had as yet in my life never before experienced complete silence before. It was like the world and stopped for me and I was waiting for God to speak to me. Then just as sudden as there was silence it was broken by a dog barking in the background and a jet flying overhead.

Another moment of silence was when I was hiking with my wife in Zion National Park. We were going on a trail in the western part of the park where there was no one and we were the only ones on the trail. Suddenly we came to an opening of a canyon area that had narrows below us and we stopped for a moment to take in the view. At that moment, I looked at my wife and whispered to her to listen. We both waited and listened for a couple of minutes while we experienced total silence. It was another treasured moment.

The last time I had experienced total silence was when I went on a scout summer came at Boulder Mountain in southern Utah. Boulder Mountain is a plateau that is over ten thousand feet tall which lies a vast wilderness area that offers a lot of places to camp for scouts. We had found a nice place and I had set up my tent a ways from everyone else so that I would not be bothered by anyone else. It was early in the morning when I woke and found that it was completely quiet not even crickets were making a noise. At over ten thousand feet above sea level it does get chilly in the morning even during the summer, and so there is not a lot of creatures out and about. I attempted to hold completely still so that I could experience the quietness of the area, but eventually I broke the silence with me moving around in my sleeping bag.

The silence in nature is one of the things that I believe is essential in learning when it comes to the mind and how the mind works and how it relates to ADHD. You see when your mind is busy it is anything but silent. I know that at times my mind is like being at a concert, or a subway station during the busiest time of the commute. It can get very noisy in there even though there is no noise audible to the ears. Then the mind is so noisy it becomes very difficult to communicate to other parts of the body and send messages to other parts of the brain to process information and to come up with good reasoning and problem solving ideas. This is why it is so important to be able to quiet the mind and allow your brain to clear up and allow thoughts to be able to surface and be processed.

Nature is a great place to be able to quiet the mind and be able to allow it to think more clearly. If you mind that you are starting to lose your mind or your child's behavior is off the wall, so for a hike or at least a walk to a park and just take the time to be mindful and experience the present moment of being in nature. I find it comforting to watch little children as they walk along the sidewalk and take the time to notice all of the ants, caterpillars, and plants along the journey. As adults we often forget what it is like to live in the moment and to take the time to see the details in things. This not only calms the mind it allows you to be able to think better and process things better in your mind.

I am continually amazed at how there is a change in young people including my daughter when we go for a hike in the mountains. The change is immediate and profound in their demeanor and countenance as they start to open up to the natural that surrounds them. You don't even have to go for a long hike for it to have a profound influence on the attitude and behavior of the child. It also has a large influence on adults as well, especially if they allow themselves to experience nature and live in the moment.

There are a lot of things you can do with nature and the outdoors that will help with ADHD. You can just take a walk each night around the block or to your favorite park instead of watching television. You can go for a hike once a week along a river, or in the mountains and get into bird watching, or just looking for signs of animals. You do not have to go far to experience the magic of nature, it might be as close as your backyard.

In many of the places I have lived there have been a host of different wild animals that have been living around our house. In one place we have a bird refuge that was only a couple of blocks away that we were able to see a variety of birds including several bald eagles when they were migrating north. We also saw several other animals like raccoons that were in a tree huddled together in a tree.

By taking the time to experience nature and to witness the beauty of the things around you, it allows your mind to be able to make calm direct connects that allow you to be able to think better. Just hiking in the mountains and seeing a large bull moose next to the trail watch my every move standing like a statue, I felt like I was the insignificant creature on the earth, and the moose was the superior of me both in physical stature and mind. Even though many wild animals do not live that long, they have learned the secrets of life and know how to enjoy it.

Chapter Thirteen: Living with ADHD in school

School can be a nightmare for someone who has
ADHD, because it requires a focused mind and one in
which keeps pace with the teacher. There has been a lot of
progress in schools these days in the handling of students
with ADHD and the many accommodations schools can
give to students who need a little extra help. But all of the
help in the world will not work if the child is unwilling to
learn in school.

The first step when it comes to learning in school is
a positive attitude and a willingness for the child to want to
learn the subject. It is impossible to teach someone who
does not want to learn. There needs to be a positive
atmosphere at school without the stress of bullying, gangs,
and the fear of being at school. The curriculum needs to be
simple yet stimulating enough to interest the children
enough to want to be there and learn the material.

I have seen too many times children that have given
up, because of the lack of support at home, the constant
failure at school, and getting in trouble at school on a
frequent basis. For many students they do not know how to
be successful in school, because they only know how to be
the class clown and failing classes. There becomes a pattern
that immerges often when a child starts to act out in school
and gets lower grades. At first the teachers and the school
are able to work with the child and the parents, but
eventually the child gets further behind in his schoolwork
and his grades begin to slip and the behavior along with it.

In the elementary years this is subtle enough that
there may not be a lot of intervention taking place, and the
child begins to slip through the system. It is by far better to
treat children with ADHD in elementary than when they
get older, however, some students do not show the signs
until later, and there is just something about children in

elementary that people seem to think that they are not able to take on responsibility for their actions.

I do think it is ironic that we are expecting children these days to learn more information and do high level math than I ever thought about when I was going through school, and yet we have nothing in place for the children who fall behind in learning the skills, and do not hold them accountable for learning those skills. If children are not held accountable for learning important skills in school then how are they able to see the worth of school later on when they are struggling to pass their math classes when the classes before did not really count.

It doesn't take children long to figure out that they can just sit around at school and do nothing causing trouble and nothing will happen to them and they can be with their friends through high school, and if they do not graduate it would not matter to them. As parents we need to hold our children accountable for their schoolwork and passing their classes. Teachers and schools need to develop a plan that holds students accountable for not learning the skills they need in school, and for their behavior.

Student pick up on things at school really fast, especially when they are in a position where the same things happen year after year. A child will not change if she is subject to the same things year after year. So if she starts to fail and get into trouble each year, she will fall into that role and continue to fail and get into trouble until something is done differently and unfortunately it is often too late.

This is why a lot of children struggle through school and when they graduate or don't graduate from high school life slaps them in the face and tells them that they now have this mountain of responsibility to take care of a family or attempt to get a good job in order to pay bills, or even finds themselves in a depressed state of living. Suicide rate is the highest among 13 to 25 year olds because of this cycle of abuse.

If you are a parent with a child that has ADHD make sure that you give him your full support and not just encourage success in school demand it and hold him accountable for his actions. Volunteer at the school and make sure that the school has the proper atmosphere that will help him succeed. Talk with teachers and develop plans and strategies to help him do better in his classes. Then make sure he is on an ADHD management plan that includes medical treatment, diet, exercise, mindfulness, and meditation. You can also get him involved in sports, scouts, and other things he might be interested in to fill his time and be able to discipline his mind and body.

Many children with ADHD feel isolated and alone at school except for when they find a friend who is in the same place as she is with ADHD. Have your child get involved in school activities and encourage him to get good friends. It is important that he has good friends and not friends who will end up getting him in trouble. It is too often the case that children at school will hang out with other children who are having the same problems and they will feed off of each other the poor behavior, and when there are several of them in the same class it causes chaos in the classroom and a headache for the teacher.

What happens is that the students know in their minds that they will not pass their classes and what they value the most is to impress other students especially their friends who are in the same boat as they are. This means that they will act out in class to impress their friends who are in class. When they are taken one by one out of the class and have to talk to the teacher or the principal the children are completely different. So it is possible that some of the students who have more severe form of ADHD and have a hard time controlling it, will need a classroom where they are independently working on assignments with one on one instruction taking place with the teacher or the student.

ADHD may lead to poor test scores with a student unable to read the test and understand the questions. She might get distracted during the test and be thinking about their friends she can text, or meeting a boy after school with her friends. In any case she will have a difficult time taking test especially standardized ones that require more focused thinking on the questions. She will know that she doesn't do well on tests and will eventually just give up on all such tests, especially since she might not be accountable for the test. So every time she is get a test she just goes through and guesses on the questions and spending the rest of the time doing other things she likes to do like working on her artwork.

In order for children with ADHD to be successful during tests, they need to be given several accommodations such as having the test read to them, learning the vocabulary that will be on the test, and being able to have extra time to finish the test. Students need the time to be able to process each question and to be able to think through the possible answers.

When I went through school, I would try to do my best on some of the tests, but it was difficult so I realized I was not going to do very well on the tests. I then began to just guess on all of the questions and be able to spend the rest of the time just daydreaming about things I wanted to do when I got home from school. I had developed this habit of just guessing on tests that I had a hard time when I went to college to take the tests, especially the ACT and the GRE which I did not do so well on. But then I realized that I could study for the test, only when I did take the test and knew the answers to the questions, I did not have enough time to finish the test and fell short every time I took the test. I knew that if I just had enough time, I would be able to finish the test and do a good job of it.

Remaining still for a long period of time for students with ADHD can be a horrible experience. Just think of spending hours in front of a computer screen doing research and typing away working on a paper that is due the next day. It can be a nightmare, and the longer it takes you to do it the longer it will take you because your mind starts to go insane. This is what sitting in a classroom listening to a teacher talk is like. The mind of someone with ADHD is racing back and forth and needs a task to do or it goes crazy, this is why some children while they are in school will do some crazy things in class and get in trouble for it. The worst part of it is the acting out ends up being reinforced instead of a negative consequence, because the acting out does gets the student exactly what he wants and that is escape from the classroom, and might even get the sympathy or admiration of his peers as well.

I hate it when it gets night, partly because I have to get up early in the morning, but also because of my several years of night classes, and it was not just night classes, it was the sitting and attempting to listen for three hours straight of the instructor going over the material. I learned very little during those night classes except that it made be hate the night, and how sitting in a class for three hours is just about the worst thing in the world. I have had classes or seminars that have lasted eight hours with short fifteen minute breaks and a half an hour for lunch, but it was torture to be there especially if it was all seat time.

The seat time is the worst, even if the instructor or lecturer is entertaining and is very good at what she does, it is torture to be in a chair for that long of time. It is the wilderness first responder classes that I enjoy the most and do the best in, and learn the most from. In the first responder classes we do not have a lot of seat time, we get up and move around and do scenarios in the hallways, on the floor, and outside even if it is raining, snowing, hot, or cold. On my initial course we even went into the mountains and hiked to a spot for the instruction. I have to recertify every two years, and look forward for each one. I can also remember the instructors as well as the material that was taught in the classes. If only all classes were taught like this.

This brings me back to schools and children with ADHD in schools. If students have great elementary teachers who do a lot of interactive things throughout the day all of her students will do well in her class and she will not have any problems with discipline in her class. This means art projects, using manipulatives in math, and acting out history through stories, and going outside for science to investigate insects around the school. If the teacher happens to have the students do a lot of seat time during the day he will have a hard time controlling his students.

Children with ADHD even if they do not cause a lot of trouble in class have a hard time with just sitting for a long period of time, and it is hard for them to think and learn. I know that my daughter might be watching a movie for several hours and not be to hyperactive, but she is not learning anything from the movie and she cannot stay in one spot, but moves around in several different spots. If I am there with her watching the movie she comes over and bugs me the entire time we are watching the movie. Even at night when she is sleeping she has to move around in her bed and cannot stay in one spot.

I am the same way, where I have to be moving around and doing different things or my attention is gone and I have a hard time listening and concentrating on things. I have recently started to do what I see a lot of other adults do including my father which is taking micro naps during instruction. In church, faculty meetings, and seminars if I am not busy writing down notes, which in many cases are not related to the topic being discussed then I start taking micro naps where I will fall into a dream for a few minutes and then wake up again to listen to the speaker and then fall back asleep. I have seen a lot of other people do this, it could a combination of having ADHD, and age.

It is hard not to be tired throughout the day when your mind is going a million miles a second thinking about everything under the sun. This will take a toll in the form of fatigue and for those of us to have to remain seated and do not have the option of misbehaving or escaping we find ways of other distraction like texting, note taking, or taking micro naps. I am convinced that a lot of the new technology in part was made to address this problem especially with adults who need to have a distraction when they are in the midst of something they perceive as being boring.

In an opening institute of teachers, the superintendent spoke for a couple of hours with a power point. I could tell he had put some thought and effort into what he was talking about and thought it was important for the teacher to learn about. He was an average speaker and the presentation was okay, but the thing I noticed was that there were several teachers who were texting and many who were doing things on their ipad. At first I was one of those teachers using his ipad to attempt to not be bored and fall asleep. I gave up on the ipad getting bored with it, and was just about to start having my micro naps when I forced myself to remain alert and attentive for another thirty minutes. But I was amazed at how many people were not really listening to the message, and would not get anything out of it.

Children go from the elementary setting where they are with one teacher, and the teacher goes over many different subjects throughout the day ranging from math and science, to language arts and social studies. The teacher will also go over art, music, and several other active things with students throughout the day. Also students get a morning and afternoon recess plus lunch. They then are moved up to middle school where they have several teachers, no recess, and have a lot of seat time. For some students the only time they get out of their seats is when they move from one class to the next.

In some high schools their classes may even be 90 minutes long and for most classes it requires a lot of seat time. Many students especially those with ADHD go crazy in this type of environment with no outlet for their built up frustrations. Give them the added stress of tests, trying to belong in school and fitting in with their peers, and it leads into a formula for disaster. Students with ADHD need a lot of hands on work, group work, and work that involves movement and action. A teacher who is having trouble with a hyperactive student might assign that student as the class helper or president where his job is to get out of his seat, pass out papers, pencils helping other children. It can be a very enlightening thing for both the teacher and the student when this occurs.

So when it comes to school for those suffering from ADHD it is important for them to have a comprehensive management plan in place, along with accommodations at school to help him to do the best he can in his classes. Those accommodations might be to have some extra time on tests, being able to get out of his seat and take a short time walking around the class helping other students, and making sure he has a PE class to help him get rid of some of his built up stress for the day.

Many students with ADHD have the potential to do amazing things at school. They can get good grades including straight As, and can be involved in sports and other extracurricular activities. Once they are able to control and manage their ADHD and understand how it works in their lives they are able to out achieve those students who do not have ADHD and are able to do this because their minds are supercharged capable of doing greater things than an average students if they are able to control their ADHD and be able to focus on the important things in school.

Chapter Fourteen: ADHD at Home

I remember having a hard time with my father growing up, and one of my older sisters had an even harder time with him and they got into several shouting matches. Now I often have conflict with my daughter over things. Living with ADHD at home can be hard especially when there are more than one person who has ADHD. The two people in the family will tend to but heads too often and disagree on a lot of things especially if it is a child and parent. The biggest part of the battle is to find common ground and be able to work with each other.

Siblings with ADHD might have a fight over several things and an ongoing rivalry where they have to compete over everything they do. They may tease each other relentlessly to the point of bullying and abuse. This could cause a great deal of stress for parents. But there is hope and a lot of things that can be done at home to make it a great deal more pleasant.

Not all children with ADHD act out at home, some of them just have a hard time on concentrating on things at school and are able to function normally at home, while others have problems at home as well. This might be where they are unable to do chores because they are too distracted by other things going on around them, especially if they are busy with another sibling. It can be a battle every day for them to complete their homework and to be able to do the things that they are expected to do.

Just like what has been talked about before in this book it is important that the child follows closely a management plan at home just like he did while he was at school, and he has to understand just how important it is to be able to follow that plan at home as well as when he is at school. This could include a well balanced healthy diet, exercise and being active, the use of medications, mindfulness, and meditation.

Unlike school as parents and family members they are able to have more control over what happens then at school. Yet the home can also be a very difficult place to be able to manage ADHD, because everyone might be doing their own thing and too busy to worry about Tim who comes home goes to his room and plays video games the rest of the day or texts his friends until one o'clock in the morning. His parents are both working and when they are home they are busy with other things around the house that they do not notice what Tim is doing until it becomes too late and something bad starts to happen like his grades start to slip or he gets into trouble.

Many homes become organized chaos where the parents are just able to fed the kids and get them to bed, but everything in between is lost. Even being educators my wife and I have had a difficult time raising our daughter, partly because when I get home from school, I am tired and have several things on my mind that I have to do, that I do not have the time or effort to encourage and help my daughter with her homework, and because I am stressed I do not want to deal with the added stress of my daughter getting into a fight we me, so I do what any sensible parent will do, I allow her to be absorbed by the television which is a perfect babysitter to help me focus on some work I have to do, or helps me to get rid of some stress from the day.

A lot of it boils down to priorities and forcing ourselves to change our lifestyles to help not only use control our ADHD, but to control that of our children as well. If we allow our children to do what they want when they are away from school and do not keep them on a management plan they will not learn about responsibility and being able to control their ADHD in other areas of their life.

I know personally that if I take a vacation from my management plan my life starts to waste away before my eyes. I used to do this when I was younger, that I would take a break from controlling my ADHD on the weekends and ended up wasting two days every week doing nothing constructive. I noticed that when I took a break on the weekend it was harder for me to get back into doing things on Monday for school. This is one argument some experts in education have when it comes to breaks in school such as summer break. They say that students are not able to retain as much learning from the year and when they start back up in the fall they need to catch up on what they lost during the summer. This is where the year round school movement came about.

I am not advocating year round school, but it is important to engage children in the summer time academically as well as physically so that they are able to retain more of their learning. This is where summer school and many other summer camps come into play. It is important for children to have during the summer so that they have something they are actively involved in something. They also need to have physical activity. The physical activities could be something as simple as taking walk to a park, or being able to take hikes or go camping.

Life at home has a hug influence over a child's development and outcome in life, especially if they have learning challenges like ADHD and have a hard time functioning in school and in situations which demand their attention. It can be very difficult to talk with a child with ADHD when he is stressed out or in the process of doing something else, it is hard for him to switch off and pay attention to the talk, and this will often lead into an argument instead of a rational discussion.

It is best to allow the child some freedom of expression to some extend in the sense that they are able to express their opinion and their rational for what they are doing or for something they do not want to do. You can even encourage her to resolve the conflict or solve the problem. Instead of telling her she needs to clean her room everyday and giving her ultimatums with punishments, you might say, "It is really important for you to clean your room everyday because it could lead to getting bugs and diseases in your room and then you could get sick, I am sure you can come up with a way to solve that problem." Then you can follow up once every few days with an emphasis that she needs to solve the problem.

We often are our own worst enemy when it comes to dealing with other people, especially when we have ADHD and it is hard to focus on others when we are caught up attempting to focus on what is happing to us. Instead of fighting with our children or others, and spending a lot of time trying to force them to do things we want them to do, we need to give them the responsibility and allow natural consequences to take place. There needs to be an element of guidance and mentorship taking place, but for most situations our children will be able to figure things out for themselves and they will have learned so much more than to have forced them to do something they do not want to do and then punishing them which makes them hate you, and end up doing the task yourself.

I remember my father getting upset with me for not doing my chores in his timetable and not doing them according to his standards. I was always trying to come up with a system of doing things that worked for me, but my father had in his mind how things should have been done, so there was often arguments over the things I was suppose to do. As an example, I would come home from school and do homework, exercise, watch television and several other things. It was my responsibility to empty the garbage. I would come home and do my other tasks and then I planned on emptying the garbage, and I did it on certain days of the week. Well my father would expect that the garbage would be empty all of the time, and would get upset with me if he saw a garbage can half fun and would yell at me for not emptying the garbage. I was too scared to explain to him the system I had and knew he would not have listen to me and would tell me his system.

Having an active creative mind can cause a lot of problems and conflict with others who have a set narrow mind about doing things. We tend to in society conform our children into molds we want them to be, but instead we should encourage creativity and the use of their imagination taking simple tasks like emptying the garbage and seeing it as a challenge in order for them to be able to use their thinking process for something good. The crazy ideas from someone with ADHD may not always work, but when they do it is near genius.

I have come up with a lot of ideas, but did not have the resources to set them in place. Long before cell phones have become so popular and have everything on them, I thought of having a watch that did everything. So think of everything that cell phones can now do on a watch. Personally I would rather have everything on a watch instead of a phone, because with phones you have to carry it around and there is a greater chance of losing it or breaking it than if it was on your wrist. With the technology we have today, it could be possible to do a watch like this with it being small enough to be able to be placed on your wrist.

The idea came to me in a dream where I had such a watch in the dream and was walking around on a college campus talking to someone on my watch using it as a phone and it was a video conference call where I could see the person and the person could see me. I also have a fully functioning computer on my wrist watch as well. The great thing about this idea was that I had come up with it in the 1990s when such an idea was only in science fiction and spy movies.

How can people come up with great ideas if their families teach them not to think for themselves and to just do as told? There are times when children need to do exactly what their parents tell them to do when there is an emergency or a high need to get something done right away. The rest of the time children need to be given the responsibility to solve their own problems with the help and encouragement of their parents.

This does not mean that children are not disciplined and they are allowed to run around the house doing what they want to do. It means that they should be allowed to be imaginative problem solvers, and that parents will not only encourage this, but push a little. Learning takes place when you do something that is difficult that challenges you both physically and mentally. If we take away this then there is little learning taking place.

I know of father who when they come on a scout campout do everything for their son. The scouts are suppose to be able to know how to set up a tent, cook their meals, and many other outdoor skills. Yet when the fathers come they are the ones setting up the tent, and cooking the meals. It is one thing to show how to do something and assist in doing it and another one to do it without any help from your son. I almost laugh and at the same time cry when I see the fathers setting up the tents and getting the food ready for dinner, and the boys are out playing soccer. Many of these boys are unable to learn how to do these things until their father lets go and has his son do these things, or that the father is unable to go to scout camp and the boy is forced into a situation where he has to learn to do these things on his own with other boys who need to learn it as well.

It can be amazing to see how the scouts are able to learn things on their own if they are left to it. But they are just as eager to let others do the job for them. It is those boys whose father always helps them, who stand around and puts forth little effort in helping set up the tent and cook the dinner allowing the other boys to do it for him. The boys whose fathers allow their sons to do these things on their own who are the ones who take charge and start to set up the tent and then come over to cook the meal while the other boys stand around or go off to play.

The same holds true in all aspects of life. You cannot do things for your children, they must learn to do them on their own, and if they have ADHD this is the only way for them. It can be hard at times so see your child struggle with things and you are compelled to step in and do it for them. You need to have patience and allow her to do those things no matter how hard it might be, because the true learning will take place through the challenges in life.

With understanding how the ADHD mind works you should be able to understand that it is better to allow a child to work out his own problems than to do it for him or argue with him because he is not doing it the way you have always been taught or that you feel like it should be done your way. Fill your home with creativity and challenge your children allowing them to be independent thinkers and problem solvers. People with ADHD often make the best leaders because they can come up with creative ways to solve problems, the only difficulty is that they tend to run up against the opinions of others and are unable to compromise or work things out.

As a parent it is important to learn everything you can about ADHD and then teach your child who has it and develop a management plan together and spend a lot of your time creating an atmosphere at home that is free from stress that encourages creative thought and allows for personal problem solving. The atmosphere of the home needs to be warm and inviting with external stimulus such as a garden, a play area, and exercise.

The child with ADHD should be treated as a member of the family and not so much different than the rest of the children in the family. The family needs to exercise together, eat healthy meals together, take time to work on the family garden and to work together to solve problems. The right atmosphere will foster learning and help to overcome the many challenges that ADHD introduces to a family.

If you have a family doctor who has experience with ADHD, he will be able to help you in ways to make the home a better place for the child with ADHD and to work out other issues. You may even consider family counseling if there begins to be conflict in the family and you do not know what to do with your son or daughter and are sick of fighting with them. You do not want to abandon the one child for the rest of the family, but then again you do not want to allow the one child to take down the family.

Just like in the classes I teach, it only takes one child to ruin a class and make it so that no learning takes place that day. This can happen in the home as well where parents are having a hard time with their child, which leads into both of them fighting and the rest of the children are fasting as well. It can become a nightmare, and you would need professional help to get it taken care of.

Love one another as it says in the bible. The home needs to be a place of love, caring, and compassion. It also needs to be a place of gratitude, forgiveness, and patience. All of live can be learned through the family and children can prepare for when someday they have their own family. I might not have been completely prepared to have my own family, but I was taught integrity and commitment by my father and mother and a little caring and compassion as well. I then through the years had adopted things I have learn to share with my family. It can be hard at times to be patience, loving, caring, and understanding, but they are essential to the life.

I have known of families whose life bordered on neglect and abuse whose children were not doing so well and struggled with having healthy relationships and doing well in school. Because of my ADHD and shyness as I grew it was very difficult for me to have healthy relationships and I was unaware how relationships actual work. This cause a lot of depression in my life and a lot of heart ache and challenges that I had a difficult time overcoming.

Through the years I have learn a great deal about myself and others and how ADHD works. The worst a family could do would be to ignore it and attempt to just go on with life. It would be too easy for parents to ignore what is happening to their child. A boy who has ADHD hates school, and hates his parents, he doesn't like it when they tell him what to do and require him to do chores when he has so much homework to do. He comes home and instead of doing his homework, his mind is racing and his stress is building so he goes into his room closes his door and puts his head phones on and blasts rap music into his ears so that he can drown out all of the sounds around him, he doesn't want to hear. Then he turned on his television and starts to play video games so he can ignore what is happening in his life. His main goal is to completely shut himself out of the world, only he is being forced to go to school and be with his family.

The parents have given up talking with him and just allow him to be in his room alone and not participate in anything the family is doing because when he does come to a family activity such as playing games, because he just fights with the other children. He starts to get further and further away from reality and his family. His grades and other things suffer at school, and his parents finally start to wonder about their boy. Eventually the boy drops out of school and moves out to be with some of his few friends who also dropped out of school. He becomes estranged from his family and only spends his time with his friends, working at a fast food restaurant.

153

The example is something that parents dread the most, but at least he did not get into a gang or drugs, only they only see him once every few months and find that he is just drifting from on job to the next and form one group of friends to the other. He has no direction in his life and no desire to change. This is what happens if ADHD is ignored and children are allowed waste away their life.

Families give these children a place of refuge a place where they feel at peace, and are loved by others. Those living with ADHD need the support from others, and this is where the family takes the greatest role. If the family is not supportive then it becomes difficult for the child or even the adult to be able to feel like she belongs. ADHD does not have to be treated like the plague or some sort of taboo that is a bad thing, it is just an obstacle that needs to be overcome and dealt with. Families are great at overcoming things that they have to face in life, and by working together they are able to do this better than any other group of people.

Chapter Fifteen: The Martial Arts Way

I remember watching Kung Fu Theater when I was young on Sunday when the rest of my family was off doing other things. The way the kung fu masters would fly through the air and most lightening fast always amazed me. I knew that they were not actually doing it, but that I also knew that there was something special about martial arts and I also wanted to be able to defend myself, because I was teased and bullied at school.

The problem was, I did not know how to go about learning about martial arts. At the time I was not big into the library thing and did not go to the library to check out books. There was no internet, and there were not very many martial arts schools in the area. There were also very few movies out at the time that had martial arts in them. It was a strange knew thing that no one really knew what to do with.

Bruce Lee had stared in several movies and was making martial arts popular in the United States, and Chuck Norris was also starting to make a name for himself, but it was still something that was strange for most people, and to tell them that they should practice it to help them control their minds was a strange notion. The mystery of martial arts to me at least was slowly beginning to reveal itself when I started to learn more about them. I had taken a karate class at college and learn a few basic moves, but most of what I learned was on my own through books that I had bought and read.

It started out with Bruce Lee and his Toa of Jeet Kune Do. Then I studied yoga, tai chi, and several other forms looking for some of the secrets of martial arts. This was a journey that I began hoping to gain some wisdom and understanding of how martial arts could help me. Later I took taekwondo classes and got my black belt. I continue to learn more information about martial arts such as Qigong, and Aikido.

The best part of martial arts is the philosophy and the practice of self discipline. It is not about the high kicks, the board breaking, and the butt kicking. The martial arts are about being focused on the good in life and to incorporate all of your life into a single purpose of doing good to yourself and others. Those you perceive or practice martial arts to fight with the intent to hurt others has corrupted the ideal of martial arts and has lost its sense of mystery. It sickens me to see the ultimate fighting and the misuse of the martial arts among those who would promote it as a way to promote violence in society.

You can throw out the idea of martial arts as something that would promote violence or is about fighting. Sure martial arts are the science of fighting and were developed in part to defend against an enemy, but the truest essence of martial arts deals more with control and focus. Studying martial arts I found that there is a whole world of information dealing with health, healing, and harmony in life.

The origin of martial arts is a clue to its true purpose. It origin came from India in the form of yoga from the ancient sandskrit what is known as the Vedas. They describe not just exercise to perform, but an entire harmonious way of living which includes diet, and how to treat others. Yoga itself means harmony. The most basic concept taught in yoga is this concept of harmony and balance of life and to have good karma. Yoga is still practiced today in India as well as many parts of the world, and many of the original practices and beliefs still exist which is almost mindboggling to not that yoga has outlived, empires, many religions, and ideas in the world today.

There are many people in the west including doctors who are trying to understand the true nature of yoga and how it applies to medicine and life in general. Yoga has become popular because a lot of celebrities have started to do it like Madonna. With the new age movement of fitness

156

yoga is one of the most popular forms of exercise among people. This is why several people have become vegetarians and have adopted more yoga beliefs. It can get into the extreme forms of obsession for some, but you do not have to become a vegetarian, or meditate for days in the same position to be able to gain the benefits of what is the harmony of yoga.

I do not believe that extremes are necessary and in many instances can be harmful. I have adopted yoga in my life in the sense that I practice some of the poses and the breathing and meditation. I also believe in some of the beliefs such as karma and making sure that I do good in the world and know that the good will come back to me. Yoga for me is also the harmony I seek in this life, a harmony between my body, mind, and spirit. Many people are busy trying to disrupt their harmony.

ADHD is one aspect of life can be very unharmonious in nature and can disrupt a balance in the body and mind causing difficulties and challenges for those who have it. By practicing yoga you can gain greater control over ADHD and have better control in your life. It can help to control the part of ADHD that gets out of control when your mind gets all stressed out and you are unable to think and your emotions start to take over and the defense mechanisms of fight, flight, or freeze comes into play. Yoga can help to teach you to be able to have control over your thoughts and emotions thus being able to deal with stressful situations.

Yoga has also been associated with Hinduism. It is an integral part of Hinduism, however you do not have to become a Hindu in order to be able to practice it and receive of its benefits. You do not have to change any of your beliefs or change religions. You can say that it is in essence just ancient common sense. It is a series of things we should already be doing.

For those of you who think yoga is a wimpy form of exercise and you feel that it is a waste of time because there is not a lot of weight lifting or intense cardiovascular fitness taking place, just see it as a foundation for your fitness routine. It helps to ground you with proper breathing techniques, meditation to help sync the mind and body, and to maintain flexibility and endurance in the body. Even the most basic of poses or stretches can cause you to be very sore the next day. Advanced forms of yoga are not for the novices, they not only are difficult at best to perform, they do have an element of risk in them. Take care to start simple and do only a handful of poses and get your breathing technique down, and a personalized meditation routine in place.

Yoga was adopted by Buddhism through its monks and spread to China where a new form of martial arts was born. First it was transformed from yoga into qigong, and then later tai chi chuan. The monks of the Shoalin temple transformed it further into what is known as wushu or kung fu which is a system of martial arts that is as diverse as the many people in China. There are dozens of different forms of kung fu, and each has its own signature from its place of origin or family that used it.

Out of yoga and the Chinese martial arts has arisen a philosophy of harmony, balance which in china is known as the yin and yang. The practice of yoga, qigong, and tai chi are suppose to be a system to help keep your life in harmony or balance. If it is not in harmony it will be sick or in chaos. ADHD is an element of chaos that causes an imbalance in your brain as well as many other parts of your body.

Through practice of yoga, qigong, and tai chi you will be able achieve this balance which is part of meditation or being mindful. The breathing, and meditation will help to calm the mind and help to clear your thoughts which is what will help to control the effects of ADHD. It is like the

158

reset button on a computer when the computer freezes. Your mind from time to time will get overwhelmed and it will freeze and you will not be able to do anything about it at the time, becoming frustrated and even angry. But if you take the time to relax do some mindful breathing and meditate you will be able to free up your mind and think more clearly than before.

I have experienced this several times in my life and have seen the benefits of martial arts not just in my life, but in the life of many others. I cannot live a healthy life without practicing martial arts. The practice of yoga, qigong, and tai chi has helped to balance my life and keep it grounded in a foundation I can live on. Without it I would be lost and my life would be thrown into chaos.

Taekwondo taught me a lot more about life and how to control the effects of ADHD. I was able to learn more self discipline and most of all respect. Respect for my master, respect for myself, and respect for others. It takes a lot of hard work to get to the point to where you can have complete control over your life. Taekwondo can give you that control. Just like most fitness routines and sports taekwondo is a series of routines or patterns that helps to develop kicks, hand techniques, and defense techniques that will help your defend yourself. But the emphasis is not on hurting others, but that of helping you develop discipline over your body, and over your mind as well.

In any given sports or movement the mind has to form connections and those connections takes time, effort, and a lot of practice. As an example when I was young, I wanted to do well in all of the sports I played, unfortunately when I first did sports I was not very good. Later when my body and mind matured a little, I was able to be a great deal better than I was in the past. In basketball I learned how to dribble the ball and shoot the ball so that it would go into the basket. I could tell by the feel of how I shot the ball if it would go in the basket or not. The feel of shooting the basket was the main area I focused on when I practiced and I managed to become good for a time shooting three point shots, and hook shots. Only as how life goes, other interests took me away from the game and I feel into misuse. So now I would be lucky to be able to hit the basket upon my first attempt. The connections in my brain are still there only they are rusty and do not work as well as they did when I was practicing and concentrating on shooting the ball.

It is the repetition of the movements in martial arts and in particular in taekwondo that has formed several connections in my mind. The more I practice the movements the stronger the connections in my mind and the more I am able to control the thoughts in my mind and have more overall balance in my life. I can do the same things with many other things such as with juggling or playing basketball. Anything that requires repetition and practice will help to control the mind. This will help you to have a better memory and later in years in will help you continue to think more clearly.

I am beginning to learn more about other martial arts such as aikido which came from Japan. It does a lot of grappling, locks, and throws with little or no kicks or punches. The foundation of aikido is non-violent resistance, being able to defend yourself without hurting your attacker. Your intent is not to harm your attacker, just to make sure that he does not hurt you. The nature of aikido does not mean that the attacker will not be hurt, if you are thrown to the ground and your arm is being twisted you are going to get hurt. In many cases it would mean dislocations, and broken bones. But you would not intentionally harm the person, and the injuries received would not permanently injure the person.

In other martial arts you will also have a philosophy that you will not injure a person or intentionally try to harm someone to get personal gain. However, if the person is coming after you and his intent is to harm you. You will be at liberty to harm or even kill the person in defense of yourself, family, and friends. In aikido the techniques were developed to be able to defend yourself and get the other person out of commission unable to fight back. This means that the other person will be on the ground in a lot of pain.

The founder of aikido had a non-violent purpose behind his creation of aikido and taught that to his students. It is one of the martial arts that maintains its philosophy as being non-violent unlike how some martial arts are basterdized in the United States to the point that many people see martial arts as being very violent, and if you put your kid into martial arts he will turn out to be a fighter.

I have heard horror stories about a martial arts teacher who told his students to get into fights with gang members so that they would be able to I guess prove themselves as fighters and to get rid of the gangs. This is why parents will think that martial arts promotes violence. If you are looking into martial arts and getting your child into some lessons, or learning it yourself, it is important to do some checking first before you commit, and do not just look at price. You are wasting your money if you pay for lessons from a school that promotes the fighting side of martial arts.

The best qualities to look for in a martial art school is if they treat everyone with respect and teach respect in their school as well as the other martial art practices such as discipline, and perseverance. It would be good for the martial art school to be sympathetic to your concerns when it comes to ADHD, and how it will affect the lessons. Normally someone with ADHD will do well in martial arts because they are always moving around, but sometimes they may be distracted by other students and want to practice kicking or punching them instead of listening to the instructor. A good school will be able to deal with this and know how to handle students that get distracted in a way that does not intimidate or humiliate the child.

If you are seriously considering a martial arts school, it would be best to watch some of the classes first to get a feel for the school and the instructors. You do not want harsh military style instructors who bark orders the entire time, but you also do not want instructors who allow all the kids to run around kicking each other and playing around either. A good instructor is one who knows the students names, is patient with the students when they do not know how to do a move, and is firm enough to teach the students discipline.

I saw all of this where I took my taekwondo classes and was pleased with this. I was also happy with being able to learn all the things I did at the school. It was tough, but not too tough to want me to quit because I didn't like it. I enjoyed all of the classes I had attended. I also liked the testing for the belts. The testing was well organized and I was taught enough to be able to prepare for them. The testing was also just hard enough to be a challenge yet not beyond my reach to achieve it.

The martial arts have taught me a lot about life and about controlling my thoughts and my body. I would say that with martial arts I have been able to gain a greater control over my life especially my ADHD. It also lead me down the path to meditation and mindfulness something that I never even heard about until I got into martial arts and studied qigong, Buddhism, and the basic concepts of meditation in martial arts. There were many times we as a class would sit and meditate at the end of class.

There are a lot of books and DVDs out on yoga, tai chi, qigong, and other martial arts that you will be able to look at and study on your own time. Many of these are also available at your local library so it would not cost you anything to get into. There is also no cost in equipment you need to buy either. If you enroll in classes you would need to buy a uniform, and there may be other cost you would have to pay for along your journey. But with some of the martial arts like qigong you would be able to learn it on your own at your own pace and without spending any money.

Some areas offer community classes that are reasonable in price and the instructors are excellent. Many colleges and universities also offer courses in martial arts which are comparable to the private schools. If you are working on a degree you can always add an extra taekwondo or karate class to your schedule without any problems. I enjoyed the karate class I took in college.

In everything this should be about you and your child when it comes to learning anything new. It should be a personal journey of knowledge and discovery where you can gain great treasures of knowledge and unlock the hidden mysteries. If you are partaking this journey you need to allow yourself to surrender to it. If this is for your child, you need to make certain that she really wants to learn more about martial arts. A child especially one with ADHD cannot learn anything they do not want to learn. It needs to be something they are excited about and will not complain when it starts to get tough for them. You may even want to teach them a few things on your own when you learn them, or even learn some of the martial arts together as a family.

I remember that there were several families that came to classes together, and the school even had a class that was for families where it was a mix of adults and children, and a class for children. It was a neat experience for me to see all of the different people working towards a common goal to better themselves and do better in taekwondo.

Chapter Sixteen: Super Brain

In this book I have talked a lot about the challenges and limitations a person with ADHD might have and the ways to overcome them. In this chapter I would like to talk about the benefits of having ADHD. Many would believe that there are no benefits and it is just a negative condition that makes it difficult at best for someone with it to learn. But through understanding of how ADHD works and what it really is we can then look at some of the amazing things a person with ADHD can accomplish.

Some of the geniuses in history like Albert Einstein, Thomas Edison, and Alexander Graham Bell may have had ADHD because they all had a tendency to be overly active in their journey that lead to some of the most important discoveries and inventions of all time. Both Einstein and Edison had a hard time with school. Bell had a hard time sleeping at night and would often get up early and think about his inventions. They were constantly inventing or thinking about new ideas and were all very creative thinkers. Einstein thought of relativity by imagining riding on a beam of light. We will never really know if they had ADHD or not, but it doesn't really matter because we know that those with ADHD have the same qualities of those who have a genius mind.

ADHD makes it so that the brain goes very fast and the thoughts and emotions are going on very fast making it difficult for someone to focus because he is distracted by all of his thoughts and emotions. So this means that ADHD can allow a person to think faster, be creative, energetic, and if it is controlled be able to do just about anything and do it better than the average person.

I call it a super brain because it can do so many things. There are just so many things that the brain can do if it is guided and directed into the right direction. Without that proper guidance and focus there is only chaos. There are perhaps hundreds or thousands of children each year who have ADHD. It is important to remember that when the child becomes bored he will seek other things to stop the boredom. This means that some children who have ADHD will get involved with drugs, gangs, and criminal behavior. They may even rebel against their parents, or act out in school to get attention.

But if all of this energy was redirected to constructive things at both home and school it would help to overcome those challenges and give children a path to go. By channeling their behavior amazing things can happen. Some kids who are those who are overachievers have ADHD, but because they do so well in school no one considers that that might have ADHD. It is just that they somehow were able to adapt and manage their ADHD without the support of others.

It is important to find something that they love to do and to allow them to focus on it and become the expert on it. Sure the other areas in school might be important according to the school board and they are required to take those classes, but it is the ones that a child is interested in and likes will enable her to focus her extra energy on and instead of getting into trouble or hanging out with the wrong type of friends.

Do not shut down opportunities for a child to be able to learn a great deal from an area he might be interested in. It can be hard to get him interest in other things. But do not give up on him when he wants to be in a band and learn an instrument, or wants to design video games, or is big into other areas that are less exciting. Sometimes people do need a little encouragement to get involved in other things or to be able to find their path in life.

A student with ADHD might not like math, but through persistence you might be able to convince him that math is important. He might get involved in this and become a great mathematician. It just takes moving him in the right direction and the proper motivation to get any student moving in the right direction. With the ADHD super brain things can be done quicker and the material would be consumed.

My entire life I have struggled with the idea that I am stupid. I had a hard time reading things because it took me forever and still takes me forever to read a book. But once I learned that I can read books by listening to them, and that certain books that I get interested in, I can read in super lightening speed. I cannot yet read like the speed readers, and do not have a desire to read a book like they do. But I now read over 100 books a year where as it took be a year to read just one book.

In the past ten years I have learned more things that I have the twenty four years before, simply because I was dedicated to learn as much as I can and catch up to everything that I had missed out on in the past. This meant that I have done a lot of things in the past ten year including earning a M.Ed degree from a local university, getting my black belt in taekwondo, and writing dozens of books.

I am now convinced more than ever that I would consider myself a slow genius in the sense that when it comes to a test, I might not be able to complete it in the time allotted by the people in charge of the test, but if I were to have the extra time, I would be able to get most if not all of the questions right. I believe that if I am given enough time, I can solve all of the problems of the world. It has opened my eyes to the fact that I can do amazing things, because my mind acts in a certain way that allows me to be very creative and to think through problems and solve them.

I also have a lot of energy and work very hard. I can do more things before noon on any given day than some people do all week long. ADHD has not given me a lazy stupid brain, but a supercharged brain that moves faster than the speed of light and can do just about anything if I am allow to think and redirect my mind into the things I love to do. Now there are certain things that will block my mind and make it virtually impossible for me to learn such as with math. I have developed a loathing for math that has made it nearly impossible to learn. It is nearly impossible to learn something you hate and that is exactly what has happened with me. The things I love are the things that I am best at and learn the most from.

Given the proper tools a person with ADHD can do amazing things. If all of those thoughts, emotions, and connections made in the brain were focused on a single idea great things can take place. Just like how a basketball player like Michael Jordan who didn't make his high school basketball team the first time he tried out became one of the world's best players. It was because he loved the game and practiced and practiced until those connections became perfect and he was able to be a good player. It is how Einstein was able to get into physics and become consumed with ideas about time and space. It was Alexander Graham Bell who thought of sending multiple messages over the telegraph wire and then coming up with the idea of sending voice over the wires. It was Edison who failed hundreds of times in order to come up with a light bulb that worked.

If you find yourself struggling because you have ADHD, you need to find something you are first interested in and then develop it so that you are good at it, and then extend it beyond just being good to being an expert at it. When people meet me they would not think that I have ran in a marathon, I was a power lifter, I teach 9th grade students, and I have wrote several books. Since I am short they may also assume that I am not very good at basketball, or football, yet I at one time was a very good shot in basketball, and in high school I played defensive tackle on the school team.

I have met several students who have ADHD who struggle doing well in school, but when I get them into an element they are good at they shine. It could be sports or a particular subject area in school. It might be that they can just talk well with other students. I had a student who struggled in school, but when he was in my criminal justice class and had him participate in youth court he was a natural and could picture him as a really good attorney. Only he hung out with the wrong group of kids who were into gangs and fighting. When he was not with them he was just fine, and he could function well in school. He had a hard time doing his work in class, but when he sat on the panel of judges talking to his peers when he came in front of the court he did better than all of the other students.

I have had several students like this who were good at talking with others and have an enthusiasm to be social, but did not do so well academically. It only takes some guidance, discipline, and a little organization to turn this student around so that he becomes successful in school and will be able to turn that into a successful career. Yet I am amazed at how these students often fall through the cracks, they continue to follow the same pattern they have always known. Parents go beyond frustration level and give up not knowing what to do. Teachers and administrators chalk it up to that the kid is a bad kid who is unwilling to learn. He fulfills everyone's predictions about himself and becomes the failure everyone expects because it is the role that has been laid out for him.

It is this role that makes the greatest difference among children especially those with ADHD who latch on to stereotypes given to them by others who do not really know them, or a family who doesn't have high expectations. If a child is given a role as being a troublemaker from the beginning and through years in school is always getting into trouble she will not miraculously change overnight and become an angel.

The child given the role as a slacker, a student who is lazy and doesn't do his work, he will play that role and become lazy not capable of putting forth an effort to do his work, because it is expected by everyone. It may start out that he is told that he is lazy, and after being told this he starts to accept this and then when he is lazy people do not make a big deal out of it, because they believe that is the way he is, and then when he is in high school he is unable to complete assignments because he lacks the study skills and discipline to do the work.

I have fallen into the same trap on both sides. I was told I was stupid and lazy several times at home and at school. For a time I worked hard to overcome this, and then embraced it for a while thinking I was lazy and stupid. I even came up with a creative way to get out of doing things in my mind thinking that I was allergic to work and it would make me break out in hives or something. I also can up with a theory that work was bad for you and that exercise was superior and work was kind of anti-exercise that could get you injured or sick. This was why men threw out their backs and had heart attacks shoveling snow and mowing the lawn. I would do just about anything to get out of work. Only I did not realize at the time that I was just playing the role that was given to me by everyone else.

No one expected me to be a straight A student, be good at sports especially since I was short, or be good at anything. There were times of hope for me to do good at school, and pick up something like music or art that I was good at. Only I was forced into playing the clarinet that I did not want to play, and I was not dedicated enough to practice other music instruments like the guitar or piano. So I went along for years believing I would not amount to much and acting the part.

Only there was something that was suppressed often in my mind deep down that was a glimmer of hope that I would make it in something. I first wanted to be a professional singer like Elvis Presley only after recording myself sing, I gave up on that dream. Then I thought of becoming a professional football player like O.J. Simpson. This was before the famous trial. But I found that I was not very good at football either and I was too slow to be a running back. Then I adopted the dream of becoming a professional bodybuilder like Arnold. I read all of his books and watched all of his movies hoping that one day I would be just like him famous and rich.

I got up early every morning before heading off to high school and exercised. Fortunately for me the gym was right next to my high school, so I could get a better workout. The difficulty with this dream was no one shared my vision, and I went about it the wrong way. I had done my research and had done a lot in the way of exercise and started to take supplements and things. Only I went through exercising too much and going through burnout time and time again. It wasn't long before I became frustrated with the whole bodybuilding thing. At one point I got almost big enough, but I had too much fat on my body and was not about to be able to compete.

I was still following my role as an average boy who was not going to make it in life. This with my shyness prevented me from talking with other weight lifters and bodybuilders and getting into competitions which would have pushed me into the next level and then I would have been able to have built my self esteem enough for me to have gone a little further in my dream. I have always believed that you can achieve anything so long as you are willing to pay the price.

My bodybuilding dreams left me after a series of life changing events such as going on a two year mission for my church, going through college, getting married, and having a child. All of these things too precedence over my body building dream, and then soon that dream was no longer part of my life. But there was one dream I had never given up on.

The dream I had never really given up on, but had postponed several times was that of writing. Ever since I was in elementary school, I wanted to be a writer and have my name on the front cover of a book. No one every encouraged me except for my English teacher in high school who helped me become creative by writing poetry, and short stories. In the 1980s the internet, computers, and many of the things we take for granted now when it comes to a writer's world did not exist. I did not know anything about becoming a writer, or getting published. Even when I went to college at the age of 21 in 1989 I thought that I would just get a degree in English and Journalism in order to be able to become a writer. Only at the time the college which they changed to a university did not have anything that was what I wanted, so I settled for getting a degree in history because I liked history. Later I decided that I wanted to be a teacher and went into the teaching program.

I had wanted to go into P.E. or something that had to do with athletics as well, only the P.E. program did not have a lot to offer, and at the time there was nothing in recreation either. So I was just stuck with a history major and a P.E. minor. Life was giving me a lot of twists and turns that I had never expected. There were a lot of times when I had just about given up and done something really stupid, but I persisted and eventually became a teacher. Only I had never really given up my dream of writing. I had enrolled in the University to get an English journalism degree, only I got a teaching job just after that, and did not follow through with it, and then got my master's degree, married, and a child. Things just seemed to fly by.

There were other dreams I had such as getting married and having a family and having a home. It was typically the American dream, and I was finally starting to see it unfold in front of me. Only there was some unfinished business I had to do. Over the years I had learned more and more about writing and getting published, only I had not written much and what I had written was not very good. There were a few books I had submitted for publication only to get rejection letter after rejection letter. I could fill up an entire filing cabinet with rejection letters, and later emails. For a time I had stopped trying and writing. There was just something that was always missing in my life, and I could not figure it out until I started to write again and made a serious commitment to writing.

When I took the plunge, I had decided to get up at 3:00 in the morning to be able to spend a few hours a day writing. This lead to writing nearly full time each week, and I was able to produce several books from this and I started to submit manuscripts each week as well, only to get them back saying that they wouldn't publish my work. I longed to be like Nicholas Sparks or Stephen King who both get a million dollar advances for their next book, and both of them have had a lot of movies made from their books. Only I was not a very good writer and did not have anyone who was willing to spend full time editing my books and helping me polish my work for submission to publishers.

Just like in anything in life, you need to make a name for yourself in order to sale yourself, and I was a nobody who had not published anything. This gave me the idea that if no one was going to publish my work, I would do it myself. So I started a publishing company, and self published a book which cost me $3,000 dollars for a thousand books which I only sold one to a woman I knew for a discounted price. I had realized that I still was not a very good writer, and did not have enough money to publish all of the books I have written.

My maturity level had changed a lot and I am able to be able to do a lot of other things in the mean time like working on my career as a teacher. I started to develop ideas for some great stories as well as some great non-fiction books. Through all of my effort and with the technology to just put it out on the internet for people to buy on line in the form of e-books. It is a simple way to get my work out for people to buy it.

I had continued to have faith in my abilities and faith that I was so much more than the role that I was placed in for my life. In India many people are born into a caste in which they are unable to leave from during their lifetime, and it is only according to their beliefs that they would tell you that the only way to get out of a caste would b to die and be reborn into a different caste. So in other words when you were born you were given a role in society one in which you cannot change unless you die and are born into a different role.

Only we can change our roles in life and even help others to change those roles as well. My biggest regret is that I have fallen into the same mistake of others and place people into their roles in society. I have seen students in whom I would label lazy, a troublemaker, or my straight A student who doesn't do anything wrong. Unfortunately I do little in the way of helping these students change when I have so many other students to work with and I get rewarded with when I see success.

In anything in the world if you are not having any success at something you soon lose interest, patience, and compassion to help those children given the success they have for those children who need just a little push to do better in your classroom. Even with the high stakes teaching and the accountability in education today, there is built into the system that educators are told not to bother with the really low performing students and not to worry about the top students, but to spend most if not all of their time working with students in the middle. This means that those students with ADHD who are trouble makers or are doing poorly in class unless they are special education students will receive no extra help, it is left up to the parents to fill in the gaps. If it is a single parent family and the parent are busy working two jobs just to support her family she does not have enough time to help your children with school work and to encourage them to do great things.

So in other word we have to go out of our way and identify all students who are having trouble in school and change their role that they have been given so that they can start to have success in their lives. Every child in school has the potential to become great at something in their lives. If they are given a role that is low they will never be able to achieve the success they so desire, because they will not have the motivation or the faith in themselves to put forth the time and effort required to make the dream come true.

The sad truth of it is that many ADHD students are the Einsteins, Edisons, and Bells of tomorrow, and if we extinguish the fire within them and do not allow their brilliant minds to develop and learn in the area they want their super brains will never be fully realized. It takes a super brain one that can be creative, and can solve problems coming up with synergy and new ideas who is moving up in the world. I am not sure if it is a conspiracy theory or not about how the government both nationally or locally is purposefully setting up these tests and other criteria to place every child in a restrictive role in life that they are unable to break free from.

Think of it as if our society is built on competition there can only be one winner, and those in charge do not want someone young who normally has the role as being in poverty and never amounting to something, being able to compete with those who always have been good and have maintained good grades. Most societies in the world live in an economic caste system where the poor remain poor and the wealthy continue to get wealthier. But this does not have to be the case and those with ADHD can gain control over their life and shine with their talents.

It is just a matter of knowing what you are good at and work on developing your talents. Even your weaknesses are there for you to develop into strengths, and many of those weaknesses will help you to be able to get stronger, because of the challenges you have to overcome, and challenges will only help to make you stronger. Find out what you are good at and what your interests are and strive to become an expert at these things, those things are the very things you will be doing for a living later on in your life. The best part of life is to do those things you love to do. The worst part of life is getting stuck doing things you hate doing. But for some people no matter what they do they will not like what they do and it isn't what they are doing is the trouble it is their attitude. No matter what job you get, do your best at that job and have a positive attitude while you are working at that job and it will be a good experience. You may even learn a lot from the experience, especially if the job is challenging and a lot of work.

Always remember that those who have ADHD have a special gift of having a brain that works faster than normal, it is just a matter of controlling that speed that matters and being able to channel the energy of your thoughts and emotions into something constructive. This will enable you to do amazing things. It is only when you get distracted from your dreams and allow what others say about you that will cause you to falter and not achieve your dreams.

You can do anything you set your mind to and be able to focus on. Remember you do have to pay a price when it comes to getting what you so desire. You have to look at what that price will be and ask yourself if that is really what you want. If the price is too great and it means losing your family and friends or your sense of peace and comfort then you may want to look for other dreams that do not carry such a high price. You just have to look at others who have achieved the same things you so desire and wonder if it is worth it.

I remember a man who was going to a business school tell me that he did not want a job that paid a lot of money, because it would mean that he would have little time with his family. He explained that those who made the big bucks were the ones who had to travel a lot and spend a lot of time at work. It was like those who made the big money were trading time spend with their family for money. This is the same in many other areas where people can take on a second job or spend more hours at work to get more money, but they spend a lot less time with their families, and this does take its toll with the high rates of divorce in the world today. Unfortunately all those who are working longer hours and making more money are driving up the cost of living which makes it so that many other people have to work longer hours just to pay the bills.

So even though you may want to get a better job, do well in school, and make things happen. You always have to remember where you came from and who you are. Do not sacrifice the best of your life for the hope of something better. But do not allow something like ADHD to drag you down either. Constantly strive to become better than you are, but also remember your family and friends and keep them apart of your life.

Chapter Seventeen: Perseverance

Once you start on the journey of being able to live with ADHD and doing what you can to control it in your life, you need to do the next step and that is to have perseverance. You cannot simply go to a doctor and get a prescription for ADHD and then not do anything else. It is a matter of a complete management system of exercise, healthy diet, mindfulness, and meditation. It also takes a lot of perseverance, not giving up on the things that matter most to you in life.

It would be easy for a child to take medicine for ADHD, but then to allow his life to become a wreck. The medicine does not do the homework for him, nor does it force him to pay attention to his teachers or his parents or even behave like a good kid. It takes a lot of effort and work to be able to get good grades, do chores at home, and to be able to focus on the positive things in life. So when it comes to living with ADHD it does take a lot of effort and a willingness not to give up.

A student might struggle with ADHD and several other learning disorders at the same time for several years, until she grows out of them or masters them to the point she is no longer affected by them. This might mean that she will have three or five, or even ten years she has to work through the challenges. This takes a lot of perseverance in order to do this. Some who have ADHD will suffer from its distractions into adulthood and for most of their life. With the improvements in technology and the further exposure to screen time among the youth, there will be a greater influence of ADHD and it will last a lot longer through a person's life. This means that many people will have to live with it for the rest of their lives. It may mean a lifetime of commitment to managing the disorder.

There are a lot of other illnesses that are chronic that people have to live with and manage for the rest of their lives. So living with ADHD is no different than any other chronic illness that needs constant care and management. ADHD is not a life threatening illness, but it does affect the quality of your life. This will mean that the quality of life you have will be in part due to how you deal with your ADHD. You have the power to have a positive attitude and to be able to do well in everything you do in this life, or it could be that you allow ADHD to control your life and dictate the quality of your life.

I have seen this both ways, there have been students of mine who have done very well and continue to do very well in school. At times it is hard to tell if these students might have ADHD, because they do so well. Then at other times I see some students who have given up and have no hope that there life will ever change and they are condemned to a life without happiness and constant failure. Ironically some of these students are persistent at allowing ADHD to consume their lives and continually fail in their lives.

There are others who will work hard for a time and see for themselves huge strides in the management of their lives, and then they will grow tired of exercising, eating good food, meditation, and being mindful of the things around them. They will stop exercising, eating right, and doing other things that will help them in dealing with their distracting thoughts. Old habits are hard to break and it will take a lot of perseverance to overcome those habits. You will have to replace those habits with positive ones and work hard and doing your best in managing your ADHD and then to persist at controlling it.

I have had a roller coaster ride with ADHD in my life. When I was young there were times when I allowed it to distract me partly because I was depressed and did not want to worry or think about life and what was happening around me. One theory suggests that those who go through hard times in their lives may be more likely to have ADHD because the mind is stimulated from the traumatic experiences. So I am not sure if the ADHD was what was causing me to be depressed or if it was the depression that was causing me to have ADHD. In any case they both feed upon each other, causing me to go through a living hell at the time.

There were other times when I had control of my ADHD and was able to do some really great things like gets straight As for my classes in junior high, or being able to attend college and graduate, and later getting married and having a family. But these things did not come all at once. I had to wait for a long time before I could find a job, get married, have a family, and finally understand why it takes me a long time to read a book whereas other people can read a book in less than half the time it takes me.

It has taken me my entire life to be able to discover what works for me in my life and to have perseverance in dealing with my ADHD and being able to live with it and control it. The perseverance was able to allow me the time necessary to work through the challenges in my life and to overcome my weaknesses and to be able to live with ADHD. If I did not have the perseverance necessary, I would not have been able to have accomplish that which I have.

Just one school year at a time, I worked hard to pass my classes, and to fit in with the rest of the students. Even when I was teased in elementary school and had chronic depression, I got up every morning and went to school. There were very few days I missed school. I could count on one hand all of the days I missed of school from kindergarten through my senior year in high school. I was also never late to any of my classes. This was my greatest strength to just persist until I was able to accomplish what I wanted to.

I knew of several students able to do better than me in grades and was more popular than I was, but it was my perseverance that not only helped me accomplish my dreams in life, I was able to able to get noticed by other people as someone who was not going to give up. I might have not tried as often or as hard as some when it came to the things in my life, but I never really gave up on those things that were the most important in my life.

There were some things I did give up on, because of the situation and the realization that I did not need to continue to do it in my life. One such thing was football. I had a dream to play professional ball. Only I did not get a scholarship to play out of high school for a college. I then decided to attempt to walk on the team at the college I was attending. I went to the spring training camp and did just about everything that was asked of me. Yet I finally came to the conclusion that it was not what I wanted to do and it was not very important in my life, and with working part time and going to school full time it would have been nearly impossible for me to do all of that and football too. I made a decision to quit and not pursue becoming a football player. When I made the decision, I felt like it was the right one and that I should not try to attempt to play football and sacrifice the time I needed to work to pay for college and the time I needed to study for my classes and do the homework.

I have also found other things in my life that I decided not to do anymore because it was not the right time, or I was not willing to pay the price or give up something else in order to be able to follow a goal. I have also talked about giving up bodybuilding, and not becoming a musician and other things I have found would not have worked for me. Yet it was the things that mattered the most like finding someone to marry and having a child with. Getting into a career in teaching and getting my master's degree all of which was far more important than other things I wanted to do in my life.

The bottom line is that you need to find those things in your life that you feel are the most important and stick with working on to accomplish those things, to be persistent in the attempt to overcome the challenges and to move forward and do your best at what you want to do. You need to prioritize and work on those things you desire to accomplish. This might mean that if you want to go to college and receive a scholarship that you sacrifice time with friends and concentrate on doing your homework and studying for the test. It could mean that you give up watching television, and spending the hours you spend playing online video games with your friends. It means that you become dedicated to what you want to do and you encourage your friends and family to do their best and to go after their dreams as well.

You may have to wake up an hour or two earlier in the morning in order to have the extra time to work on things. It might be that you attempt to do things you have never done before in order to be able to do that which you desire. It could be that you have to face your fears to overcome things you were unable to do before. Perseverance is all about facing your fears and being able to overcome them. Wars are not won over night, even battles may take several days before they are over.

I had to face a lot of my fears in order to be able to accomplish my dreams in my life. Those fears ranged from being afraid to speak to people, to being afraid of my own abilities and not having enough faith in myself. After several years of being teased and thinking I was not very good in elementary school it took me a lot time to convince myself that I could do things and accomplish some of my dreams. It was difficult for me to begin to overcome those fears.

Fear comes from the lack of faith and love in one's life. If you lack love where you feel no one loves you, there tends to be a lot of fears that surface dealing with it and it is hard to ever feel that you can measure up to others and always wonder how other people feel about you. The lack of faith is the same thing. If you do not believe you can do something then you develop a fear of even attempting it. If you have faith that you can accomplish something then you will be able to face any fears you have and make the effort to do it. But it only is all for naught if you do not have the perseverance to continue and push forward with a willingness to stick with it. Without sticking with it you will not be able to overcome the obstacles that are placed in your path. It is a matter of hard work and not giving up on what you have started.

You need to follow through and do everything you make a commitment to do and have the integrity to do and no matter what. If you make a commitment to meet with someone then make sure that you are on time to the meeting. By making those commitments you prove to the person you are meeting with that you can be trusted and this will help you to be able to do those things you have committed to. It helps to have people on your side to help you through some of the obstacles you are faced with in your life and rely on their support. Part of perseverance is the ability to call on those people in your life who would be able to help you when an obstacle come in your direction.

There will be several times when you will want to just give up on trying anymore, but you will need to stick with it and do everything in your power to continue to do your best and overcome the obstacles in your life in order for you to achieve your dreams. Just like in exercise, you do not see any results until you have been exercising for more than a month, and then in order to improve or maintain a healthy body you need to develop a lifetime routine you can follow. Without this you will continue to fall into the same traps that caused you problems before.

Perseverance is the key to achieving what you want to achieve in this life. If you work hard long enough anything is possible. I have experienced this throughout my lifetime with all of my major dreams being fulfilled not the next day, week, or month after, but years down the road when I am refined enough to receive them. I have learned that I do not fulfill my dreams when I first want them, but when the time is right partly because I am not yet ready to receive them. So if something does not come right away you need to work hard at it and think about it as you are not yet ready to accomplish it there is something that you are still in need of learning first before you accomplish your goal.

You have probably heard that it is the journey that matters in life not the destination. This is so true in many different aspects. You will learn so much on the journey you have set for yourself, and it is how you do your journey that matters. I have found that short cuts only lead to disaster, and choosing the right path will help you make the right decisions in your life. The journey is what helps to prepare you for the destination and if you attempt to shorten the experience or catch a ride from someone else you may not appreciate the destination when you get there and you may not be prepared for what you find.

I have been on several trails in my life both mountain and desert trails. I have found that it is best to stay on the trail and to be on the right trail in order to get to the destination, and taking my time to enjoy the journey makes the destination so much more worthwhile. There are times when I am really exhausted and feel like I am not going to make it and feel like quitting, sometimes there are special moments where I see a large bull moose next to the trail staring at me, or a herd of elk grazing in a meadow. Some people feel that such places like a waterfall, or scenic area should have a road built to it so that people would not have to hike so far to it. But it is the hiking to the place that makes these places so special. Anyone can catch a ride to Old Faithful, or many other natural wonders, and there are several mountains people can drive to, but it is those natural wonders you have to hike to, are the better places because of the journey.

The journey is the perseverance that I have spoken of, and so living with ADHD you might have a desire to finish high school, go to college, get married and raise a family, or it might be that you want a good job, and be successful in the career you have chosen. The journey to get to those things will be hard for you and will require a lot of patience and understanding that you will need to learn a lot like discipline in order to be able to achieve your goals in life.

You could say that ADHD is the distracter along the journey. It could be the blister that is forming on your big toe, or the fatigue you are feeling as you hike up a mountain. It may be the small voice in your mind that is telling you that you do not need to climb the mountain or see the waterfall at the end of the trail. By learning to take care of your blisters, overcoming your fatigue and focusing on your desire and faith that you can reach the summit of the mountain will build your character and strengthen you. It will also help you to do many more things in life. Once you are able to do many of the things in your life you will be able to prepared to take the journey for others.

Through hard work and study habits in high school it can help you prepare for college. I was not ready for college when I graduated from high school partly because of my attitude, but after spending nearly two years on a church mission, I was more mature and felt more like attending college than I had done before. The time was right and I was able to finish college four years later, whereas I believe if I would have gone right after high school, I might not have been as prepared and would have dropped out never to have returned. There have been several other times when I thought I was ready for something, but time proved me wrong. It is perseverance that helped me to not just get to the destination, but to learn all I needed to know along the way.

Chapter Eighteen: Faith

As spoken of in the last chapter it is by faith that I was able to overcome my fears and accomplish my goals. In order to really understand faith you must first understand fear. It is one of those emotions that can help to protect or save your life, but it can also destroy you if you allow it to take charge. Some people have so much fear in their lives that they cannot even leave their homes without being paralyzed with fear. It can influence the decisions we make and force us to avoid doing things that can help us in the long run.

Fear is often a temporary emotion that causes both mental and physical distress. It can cause so much physical distress that it can cause someone to have a heart attack. You could literally be scared to death. Our body's natural response to fear is to increase heart rate, and adrenaline. We have what is known as the fight or flight response. I have also read about how it can cause a fight, flight, or freeze reaction so that you fight your fear, run away, or become paralyzed and freeze unable to move, speak, or think. In some cases this response can help save our lives such as running away from a wild animal, or fighting a mugger.

But in many other circumstances such as taking a test, having a job interview, or speaking to a group of people, these responses will hurt you. Think of freezing in an interview unable to speak, or running away from a pulpit at a talk, or arguing with a member of your family. All of these things will only lead to disaster and will cause some serious repercussions making it difficult at best to recover from something like running out of an important speech you were suppose to give to people at your work. I do not think your boss would be sympathetic to an explanation that you give indicating that you were too scared to give the talk.

Living with ADHD, I have had a lot of fears in my life. The fears arise from feelings of inadequacy. With having difficulty reading, and concentrating on things, I developed a fear that I was stupid and not capable of finishing school. It was not only the fear I had placed in my mind, it was reinforced by my family and those at school, so that the fear became a real fear to me that caused me to be depressed and have a really hard time for several years. It is only as an adult that I realized that this fear was false and it was based on false assumptions. Just because I had a hard time reading and struggled at school did not indicate that I was stupid, or that I couldn't accomplish many things in my life. Eventually I proved myself and others wrong and was able to do things that I had never thought I was able to do.

It was also the experiences in my life that lead to my greatest fears. I was teased in elementary school, and did not have any true friends I enjoyed being around. There were some friends in my neighborhood, but I did not enjoy spending time with them, and they would end up playing cruel jokes on me, like playing kick the can where I was it, but instead of hiding for me to find them, they took off to play something else, leaving me playing kick the can without anyone to find.

My family life was no better with older sisters who would tease me, and my father who would constantly get upset with me for doing things that I thought was the right thing to do. I had develops many fears in regards to people. Such as a fear that no one liked me, and if no one likes me, no one would want to ever have a relationship with me and I would not have any friends. I feared talking to people, believing that they would not like what I would have to say, and I was bound to always say the wrong thing to people.

I was more afraid of my own shadow than anything else. I remember thinking about how much I hated myself. I did not like the fact that I was short, that I was shy, and I was not good at anything. Even those things I thought I was good at, I found out later that I was not very good at after all. But the irony of thinking I was not good at those things was that I could have been good at those things if I would have just put the time and effort into them. Instead of being scared of people making fun of me and saying that I was no good, I should have just pushed that to the side and went about proving them wrong by becoming good at those things. But at the time I had no faith only fear and I allowed the fear to control my life and force me to abandon some of the things I was interested in and thought that I was good at like music. Even though I did not play a musical instrument and could not sing, I could have taken music lessons and voice lessons which in retrospective would have helped me tremendously in overcoming my shyness and would have built up my confidence in my abilities. It wasn't until later that I did take clarinet and guitar lessons but that was at a time when I had other things going on and had already convinced myself I was not going to be good at music.

In elementary school, I also was interested in art, and one year entered the reflections contest, only the entry I entered my teacher thought that the bald eagle I had drawn didn't look very good so she changed it and drew what she thought was a better one. This upset me, because it was not my work, but hers and the fact she did not like what I drew devastated me. I ended up getting an honorable mention for my drawing, but it was not mine so I did not think of it as very much of a recognition. I did not enter any more reflection contests, and did not do much in the way of art until I was in junior high and high school, and did not embrace it until later in my life.

With every let down it drove me further into depression, and I hated myself even more. When you find out you are not good at anything and you cannot do anything to improve your situation everything becomes hopeless and fear becomes the ultimate companion. It is what I would see hell is like. Just think of living in a place where you have no purpose, mission, and you are not good at anything, and you have no one to encourage you. It quickly becomes a very scary place, one that is far worse than just about anything I can ever imagine. Viktor Frankl in *Man's Search for Meaning* spoke of how those with hope in the death camps during World War II survived longer than those without hope. I can honestly say that being in a death camp with hope is a better place to be than to be a child trying to survive childhood without hope.

It pains me to see these children in my classroom who have given up on life. I want to just reach out and shake them awake to the knowledge that they can do anything and they can become anyone they want to be. It would be a perfect world if we could go around and hand out hope to people. Hope leads to faith.

How can you drive out your fears and gain hope and then eventually faith? Fear is one of the most powerful emotions there is. It can cause people to be irrational and do things they would not even dream of. Fear is the number one killer for people who get lost in the wilderness. People panic and cannot think rationally to be able to get adequate shelter, stay in one place so that people can find them. Rescuers find people who have died next to a river from dehydration, die from exposure to the elements when there are trees and plenty of brush to make a shelter and build a fire. Hunters end up dying of starvation when they have a rifle and plenty of ammunition. Panic and fear is what causes the death of a lot of people in emergency situations. It is the calm behavior of paramedics and emergency personnel who are able to come on a scene of chaos and restore order.

In order to overcome fear you need to first understand it. Fear is as complex as it is powerful. A fear could be a real fear such as being in a home that is on fire, your fear would be telling you that you need to evacuate the home, which would save your life. It could be a simple irrational fear that you are going to fail a test in your math class when you are good at math and have studied for the test. The fear could be based on false information or previous experiences you have experienced such as being stung by a bee, you then have a fear of bees to the point you panic if you see a bee near you. Some of the greatest fears are the fear of snakes, animals, and insects that can bit you. People can imagine what it might be like to run into a rattlesnake and have it bit you, because of all of the movies you have scene with images of rattlesnakes striking.

Another powerful fear is that of public speaking and people in general. This is because we are very social and all of our emotions reside on what others think and do in our lives. We are born wanting our parents to love us and care for us, then we start desiring the attention of our peers and wanting to be accepted by friends. Later it is that we want to be recognized for our efforts at our jobs. But on the flip side of the coin we fear that our parents will not love us or want us, we fear that we will not have any friends and our peers will not like us, we fear that we will not be accepted by other people, and we will not be recognized for our efforts at our jobs. These fears will grow if we have experiences that reinforce our fears. This might be that we give a presentation where those in the audience laugh at or say that it is too boring or did not like it. We may be teased by others, or have other people make negative comments about us.

The first thing to do it to identify the fear, and tell yourself what you are scared of and why you are scared of it, and once you have identified what the fear is and what cases the fear, you then are able to start diminishing the fear. You may never eliminate the fear from your life, but you can lessen its impact on your life. I have had a severe form of fear when it came to talking with people, but this fear has diminished greatly. I used to get really nervous to the point of being sick before talking with other people. I still get a little nervous, but I no longer get sick and I am able to do the thing that I need to do without hesitation.

The next thing you must do is to take action, and face your fears. But do not face your fears without a arsenal of weapons. The weapons you can use on fear are love, and hope. Love and hope often go hand in hand together and they will be your greatest weapons against fear. Just think of it as fear is the doubting of certainty. Love and hope is the assurance of something going to take place. We can look at it as if someone lets you know that they love and care about you, it gives you hope that you will be able to do great things. It can be amazing what the power one person can give another by just showing they care about that person. If one person can give hope to someone and can change their life, just thing what power comes from several people showing that they care for someone. This is where those students who have a loving family, friends, and teachers who care for them do so well in school.

Let's say you do not have a loving family, or friends who care about you. How do you overcome your fears? You start show that you care for other people through service and charity. You can gain hope and rewards through serving others. When you see the light go on in other people the light shines in you. One of the greatest ways to overcome fear is by loving other people and serving them. I like the Harry Potter books because it explains that it was love that his mother had that saved his life when he was an infant, and later it is the love of his friends that saves him, and ultimately it is Harry's love for other people that saves him and those around him. With each experience he had he gained greater strength over his fears and his hope grew along the way until he had sufficient faith to be able to defeat his enemies including his fears.

I have to admit it, I have had a rough life and did not know anything about facing my fears, and there were several times I allowed my fears to get the best of me. But with time I have learned several things and have been able to suppress some of my fears and face others. Ultimately it was the hope that grew inside of me that I was going to have my dreams come true, and do all that which I desire to do.

There was always a glimmer of hope in my life, but it grew when I had discovered that it is a good thing and that it is powerful enough to overcome all of my fears in my life. I have struggled for year to understand my fears and to be able to overcome them and gain the necessary hope to continue on in life. Without hope it would have been impossible for me to have faced my fears, and without it I would have been lost eventually causing my destruction.

Eventually the love and hope I had in my life turned to faith. Faith is the belief in something that cannot be seen. But it can be felt and it can be proven true in your mind through your spirit. You have probably heard about mind over matter, and the amazing things people have been able to do to control their bodies and to do great feats in life.

Many athletes including Olympic athletes will break records and become better than the previous generation in part to faith, and to a lot of hard work in training for their sports. Many people have been able to build successful businesses, have successful careers, and have great relationships with others because they have faith in their abilities and their vision for what they can accomplish.

Whenever I do something, I start out with the faith that I can accomplish it. If I start to doubt my ability fear creeps in, but it is through faith that I take action and do whatever it is I want to do. The true test of faith is not in the doing, it is in what happens after the attempt. Because the nature of life is that we all fail and often more than once, and the true test of faith would be to get up and try again. A runner may not win the race, but has won it in his heart if he did not quit and he finished the race. Almost every athlete has lost a game, a race, or an event, but has got up and worked harder for the next time she has a game, race, or event to win.

Steven King wrote several stories before he was able to have a best seller, Edison failed hundreds of times before he came up with a light bulb that would work. Many more people who are looked at being famous in history failed at things. Abraham Lincoln ran for several political offices and lost before becoming president. He did not give up the fight as president to hold the country together during the time of the civil war.

It is the confidence and faith that all will be well despite setbacks, despite failures, and despite the lack of faith of others. There is nothing you cannot do if you have enough faith to do it. You might not be able to do it the first time, or be able to convince others of your future success, but if you have sufficient enough faith you will eventually succeed. It might not be the success that you expected but it will be the success that is best for you.

Through the years of constant failure, fears, self doubt, and depression, I had some hope that I would be able to have success in my life. I have had people who have cared about me and have showed their support. See other people with hardships and helping them, I have been given hope, because I know I am not the only one who is going through fears and troubles in my life.

ADHD has made things complicated in my life and have increased some of my fears, but it has also strengthened me and has helped to toughen me enough to overcome the fears in which it had created in me. It was the one piece in my life that forced me to work harder and to make it so that I could be sufficiently strengthened to be able to have the confidence and faith necessary to do what I needed to do. It is like having a coach or trainer who pushes you to do your best when you are being trained.

I realize that ADHD did create many of my fears and made it more difficult for me to learn to read and caused me to have trouble with being able to listen to my teachers and do some of the assignments in school. But it was the single thing I need to keep me on my toes and to help me stay more focused on what I needed to do in my life.

Faith is what helped me to overcome the negative aspects of ADHD and it gave me the strength and determination to be able to move forward in my life and accomplish my dreams. Without faith, I would not have made it this far in my life. With faith, I have been able to do so much more and I have been able to have the faith in my abilities to try even when I do not succeed and fail in life my faith has allowed me to get back up again and to keep trying until I succeed. I have made a lot of mistakes in my live and will continue to make mistakes, but I know that if I keep going and have enough faith I will be able to learn from my mistakes and get past them.

Chapter Nineteen: Harmony

Living with ADHD I have learned to develop harmony or a balance in life. ADHD is anything but harmonious, because it causes distractions and makes it hard for you to think, concentrate, and focus on things around you. I had always thought that I was just bad with names, but I have found out that with my ADHD it distracts my mind just long enough that it is hard for me to take a name and put it in my long term memory, and especially when the name is not as important to me, I will forget it as soon as I hear it from a person.

Harmony is the perfect balance of things. I do not know if I will ever achieve a perfect balance in my life, it takes a lot of effort and a lot of work to just get to the point that things resemble harmony, but are not yet perfect. There are several things in life you have to juggle, and ADHD is one you do not want to have to juggle, because it causes other problems in your life, but those with it have no choice and they have to learn to live with it by juggling all of the issues with it and to develop a complete management plan.

As talked about in previous chapters in order to achieve harmony you need to be able to have a complete management plan which should include exercise, diet, meditation, mindfulness, and could include medication. It also includes developing a schedule and sticking to a routine where you have routines where you develop positive behaviors that you stick with each day in order for you to accomplish things. It is like going to school and making sure to go to every class and in a single binder keeping track of study notes and homework.

Your life will be so much more harmonious if you have a complete management plan instead of only relying on one thing to control your ADHD. It is also important to have a support teach which would include family and friends and possibly your doctor and specialists who can help support and assist you when you need the help. I am convinced that when you are able to have harmony in your home you will be able to achieve your goals as well. If you are not in harmony with your life, you will go through life struggling at every turn. The ultimate goal living with ADHD would be to achieve a sense of harmony in your life.